Plants, Food, and People

A Series of Books in Biology

Cedric I. Davern, Editor

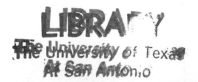

Plants, Food, and People

Maarten J. Chrispeels
University of California, San Diego

David Sadava
The Claremont Colleges

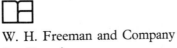

W. H. Freeman and Company
San Francisco

Cover photo courtesy of U.S.D.A.

Library of Congress Cataloging in Publication Data

Chrispeels, Maarten J   1938–
  Plants, food, and people.

  Bibliography: p.
  Includes index.
  1. Agriculture.   2. Food supply.   3. Food crops.
4. Nutrition.   5. Population.   I. Sadava, David, joint
author.   II. Title.
S495.C54   338.1′9   76-46498
ISBN 0-7167-0378-5
ISBN 0-7167-0377-7 pbk.

Printed in the United States of America

9 8 7 6 5 4 3 2 1

CONTENTS

Plants, Food, and People

CHAPTER 1 Introduction: The Problem

Too many people are hungry. Can the earth produce enough food to feed these hungry people, as well as the millions more who are born each year?

The problem of hunger is not new. It has haunted the human race throughout its history. Primitive man relied on hunting and gathering for food. Food could not always be found, and was hard to store; so starvation could occur at any time. With the coming of agriculture, when people could plant crops and keep domestic animals, the food supply became more dependable, and existence more certain, than ever before. Traditional agriculture was and is dependent on environmental factors, such as the richness of the soil, abundance of water, presence of pests, and the weather. Ancient Babylonia rose and fell with changes in the fertility of its soil. Drought caused crop failures and starvation in Egypt in 1500 B.C.; drought right now is afflicting several hundred thousand North Africans. The chronicles of famine are numerous, but their message is always the same: growing food is a precarious undertaking, highly sensitive to changes in the environment.

Famines, which are periodic hungers caused by natural disasters, have recently been overshadowed in importance by the chronic, never-ending hunger of a significant proportion of humanity. In an address delivered to the World Food Conference in Rome in 1974, U.N. Secretary-General Kurt Waldheim estimated that 800 million people, more than 20 percent of the human population, are not receiving an adequate diet, and that if food production does not increase, these people will live out the remainder of their lives nutritionally impoverished. The chronic hunger of these millions results from two facts: not only are there continually more people to feed, but some people are getting a continually larger share of what food there is.

According to anthropologists (see Table 1.1), the human population at about 8000 B.C., in the early stages of the practice of agriculture, was about 5 million. In the next 8,000 years, it grew to 250 million, and, by A.D. 1650, it had reached half a billion. The next doubling took only 200 years, and the next, to 2 billion people, was completed by 1930. The latest doubling, to 4 billion, was reached early in 1976. Thus not only is the number of people increasing, but also the rate of this increase is accelerating. As the 1970's began, the world population was increasing at the rate of 2 percent per year. If this rate is maintained, the next doubling of population, to 8 billion people, will occur within 35 years.

The population growth rate has two components: addition by birth and subtraction by death. With a high birth rate and a low death rate, the growth of a population will be high. Throughout human history, the birth rate has fluctuated somewhat, but usually changes in the death rate have had the greater effect on population growth. Thus the Black Plague, which affected much of Europe in the Middle Ages, greatly reduced the population growth in Europe for at least a century. Modern medicine has, by combatting infectious diseases, reduced the human death rate and increased the rate of population growth. Data for growth rates in various regions of the world are given in Table 1.2.

Table 1.1. Increase in human population.

Date (A.D.)	Estimated human population (millions)	Doubling time (years)
1.	250	1500
1650	500	1500
1850	1,000	200
1930	2,000	80
1976	4,000	46

Table 1.2. Growth of human populations, 1971.

Region	Births	Deaths	Net growth	Doubling time (in years)
	(per thousand people per year)			
World	34	14	20	35
Africa	47	20	27	26
Asia	38	15	23	31
North America	18	9	9	75
Latin America	38	9	29	24
Europe	18	10	8	88

In the underdeveloped areas of the world, the birth rate is high and the death rate (although high by the standards of the developed areas) is reasonably low and declining. Thus the population will continue to grow at an increasing rate as long as the birth rate remains high. In the developed countries, on the other hand, population growth is declining because the birth rate is declining. This decline in birth rate has often occurred as an area becomes technologically advanced, but the reasons for the decline are not clear. Certainly the availability and social acceptability of population-control measures (such as birth-control devices and abortion) have played a major role in the decline of births. The presence of an assured food supply and social stability may also reduce the desire for more children. Whatever the cause, the fact remains that the high birth rate in the underdeveloped countries is a prime factor in the "explosion" of the human population.

In order for the birth rate in undeveloped countries to be lowered, not only must the people have access to cheap and simple methods of birth control, but also, and most importantly, the people must *want* to use birth-control devices. Parents who are illiterate, who have an inadequate diet, who see many of their children die, who live in areas where there are few social services, often desperately want to have large families, because their children are their only hope for the future, their only assurance that someone will take care of them in their old age. Thus, where there is poverty, there are high birth rates. In general, these birth rates decline as more and more people gain access to social and economic services provided by the community.

Historically, a decline in death rates, caused by lower infant mortality and better health care, has always preceded the decline in birth rates by many years. Thus there is a period—when birth rates are still high, but death rates have already dropped—when population growth is very rapid. This period is called the *demographic transition*. Most developed countries have completed their demographic transitions, and now have both low death rates and low birth rates, resulting in a low rate of population growth. Many underdeveloped countries are now in the middle of their demographic transitions. A striking example is provided by Taiwan, which had a birth rate of 46 per thousand and a death rate of 10 per thousand in 1952. By 1972, these figures were 24 and 6, respectively. Thus the population growth rate has been halved. Many underdeveloped countries are trying to reduce the birth rate by 1 per thousand per year.

Massive programs of birth control require massive social improvements if the programs are to be successful. Education must be improved. In 1973, the U.N. estimated that about half the people in the underdeveloped countries were illiterate. Several studies have shown that as the educational level of mothers rises, there is a decrease in both the number of children they want and the number they actually have. For example, C. Miro found that, in Chile, mothers with no education averaged about 5 children, whereas those who went to elementary school averaged less than 2. A second social improvement needed for acceptance of birth control is health-care service. In the underdeveloped countries, where up to 18 percent of the infants die in their first year (the figure is 2 percent in the developed areas), parents will have many children as "insurance" against this high mortality rate. Information from China indicates that provision of adequate health care and sanitation for all people, rural and urban, has greatly helped in lowering that country's birth rate. Finally, people must be assured of an adequate food supply if the birth rate is to be reduced. In order to want fewer children, parents must be sure they can provide their children with a diet which will enable the children to live out their maximal life spans. Education and good health care are not very useful to malnourished or starving people. Whereas education and health-care delivery systems depend largely on social conditions, the ability to provide the basic necessity for life, food, depends on agriculture. Improvements in food production will make it possible to improve the diets of billions of people.

The U.N. has made projections of future population growth based on three possible scenarios (see Table 1.3). The difference between the three projections is the amount of time it will take for the population to reach a state where couples are replacing themselves only (having two children). Because the population has many more young people (who are reproducing) than older people, the reaching of replacement-level fertility will not lower the birth rate down to where it equals the death rate. This equalization will only occur many years later. The "low" projection is the most optimistic, assuming worldwide replacement-level fertility by 2020; the "high" projection assumes it will be reached around 2070; the "medium" projection

Table 1.3. U.N. population projections (in billions).

Scenario	1970	2000	2050	2150
Low	3.6	6.0	9.2	9.8
Medium	3.6	6.5	11.2	12.3
High	3.6	7.1	13.8	16.0

assumes 2045. The figures for projected populations demonstrate why the need for population control is so urgent: the longer birth-control measures are delayed, the greater will be the final population that is reached.

An increasing population places increasing pressures on the capacity of the earth to produce food. Until the first quarter of this century, the problem was not serious, since many countries had arable land which could be brought into cultivation as the population expanded. Costs of bringing new lands into cultivation were moderate, and if land was not available in the country which needed it, there was always the possibility of trading with (or conquering) those areas where land was abundant but people were few. The situation in 1975 is quite different. Many countries have all their arable land under cultivation. The vast tracts of uncultivated arable land which remain are primarily in the tropics, where costs are very high and knowledge of the area is insufficient. Population increase is now so rapid (80 million were added in 1974) that it would be extremely difficult to feed the growing numbers of people simply by expanding the land under cultivation.

Thus agriculture has turned to increasing the yield of the land, that is, the amount of food that a given area of land can produce in a certain amount of time. The transition from "area" to "yield" agriculture has been most marked in the developed countries, because increasing yield has required great technological and financial development. In the last decade, "yield" agriculture has spread to the underdeveloped countries, where it has become known as the "green revolution."

A second factor putting pressure on the world food supply is the rising affluence of the developed countries. Just as their affluence has caused the technologically advanced countries to use far more of the world's oil and minerals than would be needed merely for the survival of their people, so has their rising standard of living led to their using a disproportionate share of the world food resources. This is strikingly illustrated in Figure 1.1, which shows the relationship between per capita income and total grain consumption. Grains constitute more than half of the human diet. They can be eaten directly in the form of bread, spaghetti, rice, or sake, or consumed indirectly, after being used as animal feed. In the underdeveloped countries, each person consumes about 350 pounds of grain a year, most of it directly. In the richest countries, grain consumption is much higher, but only a fraction of the grain is eaten directly; most of it is used to produce meat and dairy products.

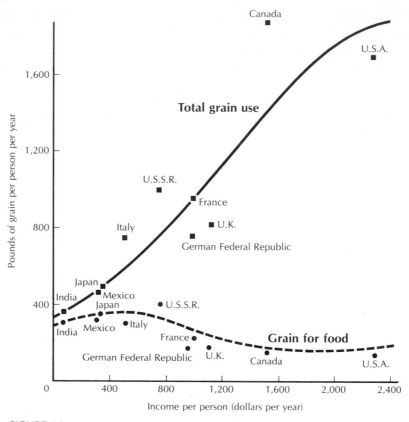

FIGURE 1.1.
Total grain consumption contrasted with grain used as food, for representative countries. (Data from F.A.O. for 1965.)

Predictions of the needs for food production must take into account the types of food that will be in demand. U.N. projections for the 1975–1985 decade indicate that, although world food demand will increase at an average rate of 2.5 percent per year, the demand for different commodities will grow at different rates. Demand for cereal grains (wheat and rice) will increase about 1.8 percent per year, but the increase in demand for beef will be 3.0 percent, for poultry 4.1 percent, and for eggs 2.7 percent. These latter demands will place increasing pressure on grain stocks, because more and more grain will be used for animal feed rather than for human food (see

Table 1.4. Consumption and projected demand for cereal grains, 1970–1985.[a]

| | Consumption 1970 | Demand 1985 | Growth rate 1970–1985 |
	(millions of metric tons)		(in percent per year)
Developed countries			
For food	160.9	166.0	0.2
For feed	373.7	506.9	2.0
Developing countries			
For food	482.6	714.1	2.7
For feed	45.3	93.9	4.8
World			
For food	643.5	880.1	2.1
For feed	419.0	600.8	2.4

[a]From F.A.O. papers presented at World Food Conference, 1974.

Table 1.4). The trend toward meat consumption is especially wasteful of grain, because the conversion of feed to meat is not efficient. In general, 4 to 6 pounds of grain (which would be 4 to 6 pounds of food if eaten directly) are needed to produce 1 pound of beef.

Thus the twin pressures of population and rising affluence are straining the capacity of the earth to produce food. The U.N. population projections show that, even if population control were instituted as quickly as possible, there would still be several billion more people sharing the earth's resources in the next century than there are today. Providing these people with an adequate diet is going to be a major challenge to man's ingenuity. In this book, we describe what the scientific bases are, and what the prospects are, for meeting this challenge.

Chapters 2 and 3 describe the nutritional needs of humans, and the central role played by crop plants in meeting these needs. The rest of the book is then devoted to a discussion of how crops are grown. First, we consider the environmental requirements for plant production: sunlight, soil, minerals, and water (Chapters 4 and 5). Next we discuss the practice of agriculture, first in terms of its origins (Chapter 6), and then as a modern science that focuses on providing the environmental requirements of the crops (Chapters 7 and 8). Improvement of the food-producing abilities of the plants themselves by breeding is considered in Chapter 9. The green revolution that resulted from the introduction of modern agricultural practices and crop strains to the underdeveloped countries is then described and its limitations discussed (Chapter 10). Finally, we examine the potential of some alternative sources of food, from fisheries to microbes (Chapter 11). We present no panaceas, for the world food problem does not lend itself to an easy solution. Rather, we hope that a presentation of the facts, problems, and potential of food production will enable the informed lay-person to understand the difficult decisions facing mankind.

CHAPTER 2

Human Nutrition

WHAT IS FOOD?

Food is any substance which provides an organism with energy and nutrients. Humans need energy to use as fuel for conscious actions, such as running or swimming, and for involuntary ones, such as heartbeat or digestion. Energy is also needed for growth and for replacing existing body tissues. The nutrients (essential amino acids, a fatty acid, vitamins, and minerals) provide the chemical building blocks for growth and tissue replacement. In addition, they are used to build the molecules which regulate and coordinate all the body's activities. The formation of every component of our tissues illustrates the need for both energy and nutrients at the same time. For example, the synthesis of hemoglobin, the protein which gives blood its typical red color, is dependent not only on the availability of the necessary building blocks—amino acids and iron—but also on the presence of energy. Thyroxine is a hormone which is synthesized in the thyroid gland and regulates the growth of the human body. Its synthesis requires an energy source, various small organic molecules, and the mineral iodine.

Not all living organisms have the same nutritional requirements. They can be either *autotrophic* or *heterotrophic,* terms that refer to different modes of nutrition. Autotrophic ("self-feeding") organisms include the plants living on land and in water and certain bacteria; they have rather simple nutritional requirements, consisting of water, carbon dioxide (CO_2), and a variety of inorganic chemicals derived from the minerals in the soil. The most unique feature of plants, the most important group of autotrophs, is that they can use light energy from the sun to provide fuel for all their energy needs. Using CO_2 from the air, water from the environment and light energy from the sun, green plants can manufacture sugar. They can then use this sugar, either immediately or after having stored it temporarily, for all their energy-requiring processes (for example, for growth and the uptake of minerals from the soil). This process of trapping the sun's energy and forming sugar is called photosynthesis. It is the key not only to all food production, but also to all life on Earth and will be discussed in Chapter 4.

Autotrophic organisms require simple inorganic chemicals, such as nitrate, phosphate, potassium, and magnesium, as nutrients. In order to be taken up by the plants, these inorganic chemicals must normally be dissolved in the water of the soil. The abundance of these nutrients in the soil plays an important role in determining the rate of plant growth and crop production. By using sugar (the product of photosynthesis), water, and the inorganic nutrients from the soil, the green plant can synthesize all the complex organic molecules it needs in order to grow and reproduce. Although both plants and animals need many of the same organic molecules to carry out their many functions, only plants can synthesize all these molecules by using only sugar and inorganic nutrients.

Heterotrophic ("other-feeding") organisms have more complex nutritional requirements. They cannot use the sun's energy directly, as can autotrophs. Heterotrophic organisms must ingest energy-rich organic molecules in order to carry out their functions. All heterotrophs, whether they eat plants (*herbivores*), animals (*carnivores*), or live on dead organic matter (*decomposers*), ultimately depend on green plants to provide them with these energy-rich organic molecules. Although some heterotrophic bacteria can grow on only an energy source (usually sugar), water, and inorganic minerals, the needs of higher animals and man are much more complex. Human beings cannot synthesize many of the organic molecules essential to their existence. They depend on plants and bacteria to synthesize these molecules for them.

For its food, an autotroph needs only:

(1) water; and
(2) minerals, including calcium, phosphorus, potassium, magnesium, iron, sulfur, nitrogen, and traces of many others.

Human beings need both of these (but more sodium, and less iron and nitrogen), and also need:

(3) a source of energy, which is normally provided by carbohydrates and fats, and sometimes by proteins;

(4) the amino acids leucine, isoleucine, lysine, methionine, phenyl-alanine, threonine, tryptophan, valine, and (for infants) arginine and histidine, which must be provided by their protein foods;

(5) the fatty acid linoleic acid, which must be provided by their fatty foods; and

(6) the vitamins A, B_1, B_2, B_6, B_{12}, C, D, E, K, and pantothenic acid, biotin, folic acid, and nicotinamide, which must be provided by various foods.

Most of these are *essential;* that is, normal growth and renewal of body tissues are impossible if any one of these is absent from the diet.

FOOD AS A SOURCE OF ENERGY

The energy and nutritive values of plants as food depend on their chemical composition. Foods vary in their ability to satisfy hunger. To understand why salted nuts are more satisfying than celery stalks, we must examine the chemical nature of our foodstuffs as well as the structure of plant cells and tissues. (A detailed discussion of nutritional biochemistry is beyond the scope of this book, however; please consult the references for this chapter listed at the end of the book for more information.)

Carbohydrates

Carbohydrates are the source of most of mankind's energy. They are abundantly present in staple foods such as wheat, rice, corn, and potatoes. They derive their name from the fact that they are composed entirely of the chemical elements carbon (C), hydrogen (H), and oxygen (O). One of the simplest carbohydrates, and the one most easily used by the human body, is glucose or grape sugar. It has the chemical formula $C_6H_{12}O_6$ and consists of a single sugar molecule (see Figure 2.1A). Sucrose (cane sugar or beet sugar) and lactose (milk sugar) are made up of two sugar molecules linked together (see Figure 2.1B). These three carbohydrates are readily soluble in water, and are easily taken up from the intestinal tract into the blood stream. As a result, they provide a source of instant energy.

A plant can convert glucose, one of the immediate products of photosynthesis, into more complex carbohydrates such as starch and cellulose. The complex carbohydrates are macromolecules (large molecules), each consisting of hundreds of individual glucose molecules linked together like

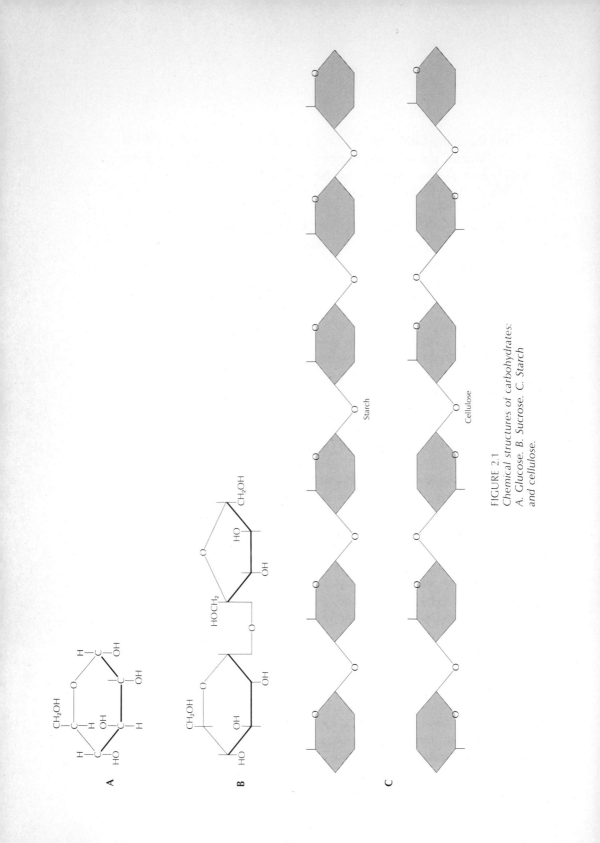

FIGURE 2.1
Chemical structures of carbohydrates:
A. Glucose. B. Sucrose. C. Starch
and cellulose.

beads on a chain (see Figure 2.1C). Starch and cellulose have different chemical and physical properties because the sugar molecules are linked together in different ways. Cellulose forms the fibrous material found in all plant tissues and is an important component of wood. Starch, on the other hand, is deposited as a food reserve by plants in specialized organs, such as seeds, roots, and tubers, to be used whenever a source of energy is needed.

Complex carbohydrates are usually not soluble in water, and they must be broken down into the simple sugars before they can be used by the human body. This breakdown is accomplished by the process of digestion. The enzymes present in saliva and digestive juices break the large molecules in food into smaller components. Humans can digest starch into glucose, but cannot digest cellulose, even though it is also made up of glucose, since they do not have the enzymes needed to digest cellulose. Humans eat a lot of cellulose; so a lot of glucose passes through the body in an unusable form. This does not mean that cellulose is without benefit for human health. Chewing, and the acids in the stomach, break the cellulose fibers into smaller pieces, which swell up as they pass through the intestinal tract, thereby increasing the bulk of the digesting food. This stimulates intestinal and bowel movements.

Some microorganisms have the enzymes needed to digest cellulose and can therefore use its glucose. Ruminant animals, such as cows, goats, and camels, have such microorganisms living in their digestive tracts, and benefit from this because the microorganisms digest the cellulose for them. Cows can therefore derive energy from grass, or even newsprint.

Lipids

Lipids, commonly known as fats or oils, are present in all organisms, being essential structural components of cells. Lipids occur in large amounts in certain animal tissues (brain, fatty tissues), in milk and eggs, and in certain seeds, such as soybeans and peanuts. Like carbohydrates, lipids are composed of the elements carbon, hydrogen, and oxygen. They are relatively small molecules, but unlike the simple sugars, they do not readily dissolve in water. This insolubility is their most important physical characteristic. Chemically they consist of a glycerol molecule ($C_3H_8O_3$) to which three fatty acids are attached. The size of the fatty acids and the number of *unsaturated* bonds (see Figure 2.2) determine the chemical and physical properties of the fat molecules. The more saturated the fatty acids and the larger the fat mol-

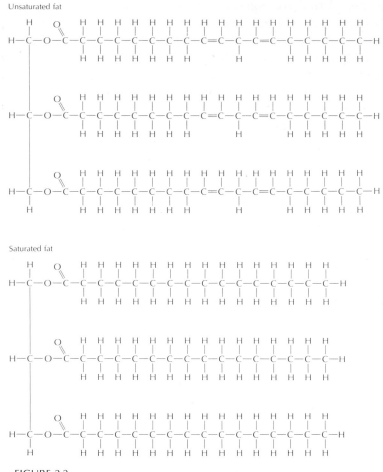

FIGURE 2.2.
Chemical structures of lipids. The fatty acids of an unsaturated fat contain less hydrogen than those in a saturated fat.

ecules, the more solid will be the fat. Fats which are liquid at room temperature are commonly called oils. Fats and oils are so similar chemically that often one can be converted into the other by a chemical process called *hydrogenation.* The manufacture of margarine from various vegetable oils (corn oil, safflower oil) is a good example of this interconversion. It has been alleged that the liquid oils—the "polyunsaturated" fats—are better for human health than the solid fats, but this claim remains controversial.

Lipids are a major source of energy for humans, but they also play an important nutritive role. Human beings need many different fatty acids to manufacture certain cellular structures, but lack the necessary chemical machinery to make at least one of the fatty acids (linoleic acid); two others have also been found to be beneficial for growth (linolenic acid and arachidonic acid). Lack of linoleic acid in the diet results in poor growth and scaliness of the skin, conditions which can be alleviated by eating fats rich in linoleic acid (most vegetable oils, except olive oil). Dietary fats also help in the absorption of certain vitamins, such as A and D, which do not dissolve in water but are soluble in fat.

Energy

Carbohydrates and lipids are the principal sources of food energy for mankind. The body can also derive energy from protein, but only when carbohydrates and fats are in short supply or when protein is in oversupply. The cells of the body obtain energy from the molecules of food by the process of respiration. But how did that energy get there, and how can we get it out?

When a plant makes glucose by photosynthesis, it uses the sun's energy; this energy is stored in the bonds linking the atoms of the glucose molecules together. When the bonds between these atoms are broken, this energy is released. Thus in photosynthesis six carbon atoms from six CO_2 molecules are linked to one another and to hydrogen and oxygen atoms to form a glucose molecule. Glucose molecules are then strung together to form starch or cellulose, or they can be converted into other molecules (fatty acids, amino acids, etc.) which are used to make lipids or proteins. When wood (which contains a large amount of cellulose) is burned, the bonds between the carbon atoms are broken, and the energy is released in the form of heat. A similar process happens in the body during respiration. Respiration is a "controlled burning": the energy is released partly as heat and partly in a chemical form which our cells use to power all their energy-requiring reactions.

The energy value (or calorie content) of foods is normally measured by burning them in a calorimeter, a device which accurately measures the amount of heat released in a combustion. The unit of energy used to express the caloric value of foods is the Calorie.* The use of one gram of carbo-

---

*A calorie is the amount of energy needed to raise the temperature of one gram of water from 14.5°C to 15.5°C. A kilocalorie or Calorie is equivalent to 1,000 calories.

hydrate, fat, and protein by the body yields 4, 9, and 4 Calories, respectively. (These values are somewhat lower than those measured by a calorimeter because foods are not completely digested and because some molecules, especially proteins, are not completely respired and broken down to CO_2 and water.)

Human needs for energy depend largely on age and activity. Young adults (age 17 to 25) need the most energy, whereas children and older people need less. Women, except when pregnant or lactating, need only about 70 percent as many calories as men, primarily because they weigh less. More than half the body's energy intake for a moderately active person of average weight (150 lbs. or 68 kilograms or kg) is used to maintain the involuntary body activities. A fasting person at rest and at 25°C needs about 1,500 Calories a day to maintain respiration, circulation, glandular activity, muscle tonus, and other basic processes. This rate of use of energy is called the basal metabolic rate.

In addition, energy is needed for food digestion (about 10 to 15 percent of the calories in the food are used for its digestion) and to compensate for heat loss, since the human body maintains a temperature of 37°C. The amount of energy used up in voluntary activities depends on the type of activity. An hour of writing, housework, or walking requires 100 to 200 Calories, whereas 700 Calories are needed for an hour of woodchopping. Finally, energy is needed for growth, tissue repair, pregnancy, and lactation. The body uses energy for many different purposes, and as a result of all these variables, caloric needs may vary from 1,800 Calories a day for a retired female clerk, to 3,200 for a young nursing mother, or to 4,600 for an adolescent boy who goes surfing regularly. In many countries recommendations for daily calorie intakes are provided by government agencies or the World Health Organization. An example of such a recommendation for different persons in tropical East Africa is shown in Table 2.1.

PROTEINS

Protein Chemistry

Protein is a major constituent of every living organism. It accounts for more than half the dry weight of the living substance (protoplasm) of most cells. Like the complex carbohydrates, proteins are composed of smaller units arranged like beads on a chain. In proteins, however, the beads

Table 2.1. Recommended daily intake of calories and protein for people in East Africa.[a]

Persons		Calories per day	Protein (grams per day)
Children,	1–2	1,000	40
	5–6	1,400	50
Girls,	11–12	2,200	65
	13–17	2,500	70
Boys,	11–12	2,000	60
	15–18	3,000	80
Women,	sedentary	1,800	55
	very active	2,500	65
	pregnant	Add 400	85
	lactating	Add 900	95
Men	sedentary	2,200	60
	very active	3,000	70

[a]From M. C. Latham, *Human Nutrition in Tropical Africa*, F.A.O. (1965), p. 243.

are amino acids, which are composed of carbon, hydrogen, oxygen, nitrogen, and sometimes sulfur. About 20 different amino acids commonly occur in proteins, and they can be arranged in any order. Most proteins contain from 100 to 1,000 amino acids, and the properties of a protein depend on the sequence of its constituent amino acids (see Figure 2.3). An ordinary cell contains more than 1,000 different proteins, each one characterized by its own sequence of amino acids.

Proteins play many important roles, as enzymes, as structural components of the cells, and as regulators of a variety of body functions. Enzymes speed up otherwise sluggish chemical reactions in the body. An example of an enzyme is amylase, which helps break the chemical bonds linking the different glucose units in a starch molecule. This enzyme is found in the saliva of humans, but it is also present in plant cells, where it has a similar role in the digestion of starch stored within the plant. Most food proteins are not enzymes, however, but are either structural proteins found in muscle cells (meat, fish) or storage proteins, such as those in plant seeds.

Plants and animals differ greatly in their ability to synthesize proteins. Plants, being autotrophic organisms, can synthesize proteins from the simple inorganic compounds carbon dioxide, water, nitrate (NO_3^-), and sulfate ($SO_4^=$). Nitrate is obtained from the soil, converted to ammonia (NH_4^+),

Tryptophan

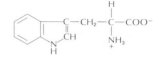

Methionine

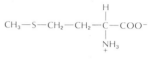

Lysine

FIGURE 2.3.
*Chemical structures of three of the 20 amino
acids found in proteins. These are three of
the essential amino acids in the human diet.*

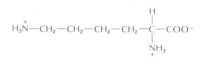

and combined with other molecules derived from photosynthesis. In this
way the plant can make all 20 amino acids and use these to form proteins.
By substituting purified amino acids for dietary proteins, nutritional biochemists have shown that the human body can synthesize only 12 of these
amino acids, but not the other eight. This was demonstrated by systematic
feeding experiments, in which one amino acid at a time was omitted from
the diet. The eight "essential" amino acids must be obtained from food,
and in sufficient quantities to satisfy the requirements of the body. If even
one essential amino acid is missing, or if there is not enough of it, we cannot
make the proteins which are essential for the proper functioning of our
bodies. Thus we must eat not only enough protein, but also the right kind
of protein, which provides us with the necessary amino acids.

The nutritional value of protein-rich foods depends not only on their
digestibility (some proteins are poorly digested), but especially on the relative abundance of the essential amino acids. Knowing which amino acids
are essential and in what proportion they should be eaten, we can assign
"protein scores" to individual foodstuffs. Human milk protein and egg pro-

tein have protein scores of 100, which means that they contain the essential amino acids in the proportions required by the human body. The amino-acid composition and protein scores for various foods are given in Table 2.2. Animal proteins generally have a higher protein score than plant proteins, because plant proteins tend to be low in the essential amino acids tryptophan, methionine, and lysine.

A marked deficiency in even one essential amino acid drastically lowers the protein score of a protein. Cornmeal, which is low in tryptophan and lysine, has a protein score of 49, and navy beans, which are low in methionine, have a protein score of 44. It is generally thought that foods with protein scores lower than 70 are unsatisfactory for growth and maintenance. This does not mean, however, that corn protein and bean protein have no nutritional value for humans. Different foods which are deficient in different amino acids can complement each other when eaten at the same meal. A meal of corn tortillas with fried beans has a much higher protein score than either foodstuff alone.

Protein in the Human Diet

Studies of human metabolism have yielded fairly accurate figures for the body's daily requirements for calories. Nutritional biochemists have similarly studied requirements for dietary protein, but have reached no

Table 2.2. Essential amino acids in selected foods. Amounts are expressed as milligrams of amino acid per gram of protein nitrogen. Egg is considered to have a perfect protein, and others are rated in comparison with it to give a protein score.[a]

Food	Iso-leucine	Leucine	Lysine	Methio-nine	Phenylal-anine	Threo-nine	Trypto-phan	Valine	Protein score
Hen's egg	393	551	436	210	358	320	93	428	100
Beef	301	507	556	169	275	287	70	313	80
Cow's milk	295	596	487	157	336	278	88	362	79
Chicken	334	460	497	157	250	248	64	318	72
Fish	299	480	569	179	245	286	70	382	70
Corn	230	783	167	120	305	225	44	303	49
Wheat	204	417	179	94	282	183	68	276	62
Rice	238	514	237	145	322	244	78	344	69
Beans	262	476	450	66	326	248	63	287	44
Soybeans	284	486	399	79	309	241	80	300	67
Potatoes	236	377	299	81	251	235	103	292	34

[a]From *F.A.O. Nutritional Study*, No. 24 (1970).

general agreement about the amount of protein needed each day. The U.S. government recommends a minimum daily protein intake of 60 to 65 grams for adult men and 55 grams for adult women. Many Americans each much more protein than this: a study of U.S. army mess halls and cafeterias revealed a daily protein consumption of 94 grams per female and 126 grams per male. The U.N. Food and Agricultural Organization (F.A.O.) has recently concluded that most adults can easily get by on 40 grams of protein a day. This figure agrees closely with the finding that the average person excretes about 30 grams of protein (or products derived from protein) each day.

Protein is excreted because body tissues undergo a continuous process of breakdown and repair. During this process, proteins are broken down into amino acids, which are then reused to make new proteins. However, this reuse is only about 80 to 90 percent efficient, and some of the amino acids are converted to urea and excreted in the urine. The feces also contain protein, derived from digestive juices and from the cells which form the lining of the intestines. These cells are continuously shed and replaced by new cells. Small losses also occur through sweat and the growing of skin, nails, and hair.

The amount of protein which is required each day depends on many variables, which may account for the discrepancy between the F.A.O. and the U.S. government recommendations. People on a high-energy diet can usually get by with less protein. The body's protein level can be maintained by a protein intake of 20 grams per day if the caloric intake is 4,000 Calories per day. The body may lose protein even when the daily protein intake is high (over 100 grams per day). This condition is usually associated with low-calorie diets. The body always satisfies its caloric needs first; if the calorie intake is low, it simply uses the protein as a source of energy rather than as a source of essential amino acids. The amount of protein the body needs is also influenced by the distribution of the protein among the three daily meals. Proteins or protein mixtures containing all the essential amino acids in the right proportions should be eaten at all three meals. The body cannot store essential amino acids for very long. Experiments have shown that growth retardation results when all the essential amino acids are not eaten simultaneously.

High muscular activity greatly increases the need of the body for energy. Many people think that such activity also increases the need for protein, that the muscle tissues become worn out and must be replaced.

This is not true. Experiments indicate that when muscular activity doubles the body's caloric requirements, it increases the need for protein by only 5 percent. College football players and other athletes often habitually eat large amounts of meat; this practice has some psychological value, but very little nutritional value.

Recent evidence shows that if a woman does not eat enough protein during pregnancy, the intellectual development of the child may be slowed down. This finding has focused renewed attention on the importance of proper nutrition during pregnancy and lactation. The growth of the fetus, especially during the final six months of development, and the production of milk require that the normal diet be supplemented with additional calories, proteins, and other nutrients (essential fatty acids, vitamins, minerals). Women who are pregnant or lactating need to increase their daily protein intake by 10 grams or 20 grams, respectively.

PROTEIN AND CALORIE MALNUTRITION

Thus far we have discussed only the number of calories and the amount of protein required by normal, healthy people. Many people do not get these required amounts: either they do not get enough food and are *undernourished;* or they do not eat the right kinds of food and are *malnourished.* We do not know (with any accuracy) how many hungry people there are, but the F.A.O. estimates the number to be around 800 million. Figure 2.4 shows that most of these people live in the underdeveloped countries of Latin America, Africa, and Asia, which are also characterized by high rates of population growth.

Hunger results largely from a maldistribution of food rather than from a lack of it. The F.A.O. estimates that, for the world as a whole, 2,270 Calories per person per day were available in 1973, a supply just about adequate to cover the needs of mankind. However, improper distribution of the available food results in overnutrition in the richer countries and undernutrition in the poorer ones. Within the underdeveloped countries, there are usually social classes or whole geographical regions which are much better off than other classes or regions. Even technologically advanced countries such as the U.S. have both rural and urban pockets of poverty and malnutrition.

A striking example of this imbalance can be found in a study made by the F.A.O. in 1970 of nutritional maldistribution in Indonesia. In one region

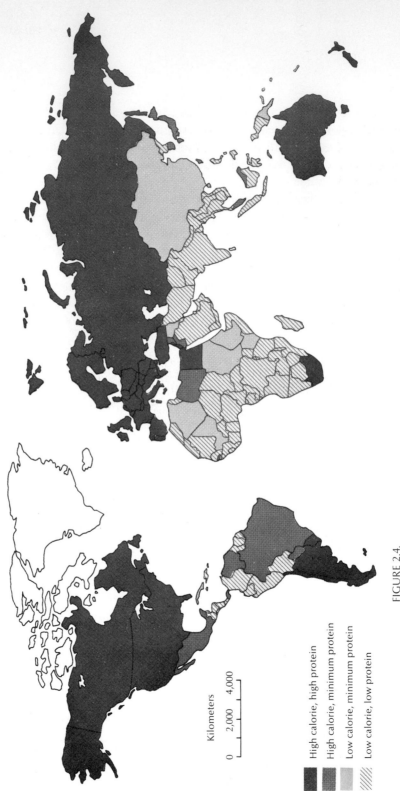

FIGURE 2.4.
The geography of hunger. (Data from F.A.O. Production Yearbook 1968.)

High calorie, high protein

High calorie, minimum protein

Low calorie, minimum protein

Low calorie, low protein

Kilometers

0   2,000   4,000

2,087 Calories per capita per day were available; in another region only 1,076 were. Similarly, the available protein varied from 46.7 grams per person per day down to 22.6 grams. The area where food was scarcest (Djokjakarta in Central Java) also had the lowest population growth rate for all the regions studied. The figures suggest that gross malnutrition can result in a decline in the birth rate. However, such severe malnutrition is not characteristic of most underdeveloped countries that have high birth rates.

People who are forced to live on diets which provide only 25 grams of plant protein and 1,100 Calories per day soon develop protein-calorie malnutrition, a combination of undernutrition and malnutrition very common among the small children of the underdeveloped countries. If intake of calories and protein drops even temporarily below what the body requires, the body will begin to metabolize its reserves. As soon as the reserves are burned up, the body begins to waste away, and working efficiency decreases. This phenomenon is illustrated clearly by the decline in efficiency of German steelworkers during the Second World War. As Figure 2.5 shows, in 1939, when workers were given 1,900 extra "work Calories," production was high. But as energy rations went down, so did steel output. Chronic undernutrition

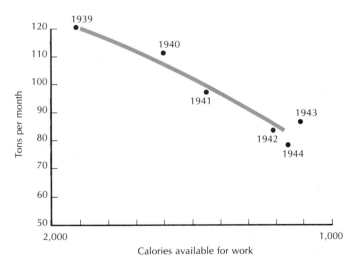

FIGURE 2.5.
Food energy and work output in a German steel factory, 1939–1944. As the calories available for work went down so did production (From F.A.O., "Nutrition and Working Efficiency," p. 15).

can also have severe psychological effects. Emotional depression and apathy are common, so common that the outsider may perceive the people as being lazy. Changes in group behavior often include a loosening of social bonds and a lessening of morale. It may not be a coincidence that those areas of the world where undernutrition is common are the same areas where political and social strife are most evident.

Protein-calorie malnutrition exerts its most devastating effects on the young. It is the most common disorder affecting small children in under-developed tropical countries. During the first few years of life, when a human being undergoes a period of rapid growth, the body must have the necessary calories, proteins, and other nutrients with which to build more tissues. If protein is not supplied, growth will not occur. This phenomenon is dramatically illustrated by an experiment in which baby rats were fed simple foods, each one receiving the same amount, but of a different food. As Figure 2.6 shows, eggs and milk, which are rich in protein, have a well-balanced amino-acid composition, and contain other nutrients, promoted rapid growth. But protein-poor foods or protein-rich foods low in certain essential amino acids did not promote growth.

Nutritionists generally recognize two different types of protein-calorie malnutrition: *nutritional marasmus* (general undernutrition) and *kwashiorkor* (protein malnutrition). Nutritional marasmus is common in infants who are weaned too early in life. From a diet of nutritious mother's milk, they are put on low-calorie, low-protein substitutes. This diet is often so deficient that the child's body wastes away, and the result may be physical stunting and permanent brain damage. These children become susceptible to infectious diseases, and their mortality rate is high. Early weaning is common in the big cities, where poor people imitate the westernized practices of the upper classes, who substitute bottle feeding for breast feeding.

Kwashiorkor (a West African word meaning "the disease the child gets when another baby is born") results from feeding a child a diet adequate in calories but low in protein, also usually after early weaning. The disease symptoms are different from those of marasmus: the body is bloated (with typical pot-bellies) because the muscles are weak and the tissues contain too much water (edema). The disease also results in arrested physical development, increased susceptibility to infection, and a high infant mortality.

The treatment of children who are suffering from protein-calorie malnutrition has given us valuable new information about the protein requirements of growing children. Children who show advanced symptoms of

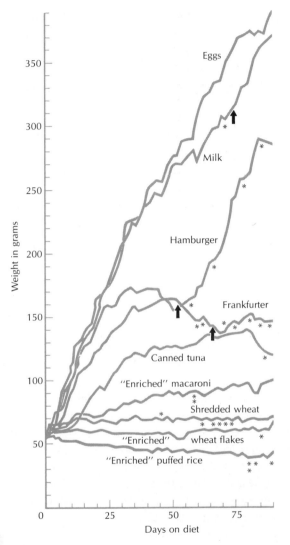

Weight in grams

350

300

250

200

150

100

50

0   25   50   75

Days on diet

Eggs

Milk

Hamburger

Frankfurter

Canned tuna

"Enriched" macaroni

Shredded wheat

"Enriched"   wheat flakes

"Enriched" puffed rice

FIGURE 2.6.
Growth of baby rats fed diets consisting of a single food. Asterisks indicate deaths of animals. Arrows indicate when diet supplements were given. Milk-fed rats were given a supplement of copper and iron. Meat-fed rats were given a supplement of minerals and vitamins. Puffed rice, wheat flakes, and macaroni were supplemented from the start with vitamins and minerals. (From R. Williams, J. Heffley, and C. Bode, "The Nutritive Values of Single Foods," Proc. Nat. Acad. Sci. U.S., *68, 1971, 2362.)*

protein-calorie malnutrition should be given diets rich in easily digestible proteins (e.g., 4.0 grams of milk protein per kilogram of body weight per day). Children who are only marginally affected by the disease can make a remarkable recovery on a "low" protein diet (e.g., 2.3 grams of vegetable protein per kilogram of body weight per day). Such a diet corresponds to a daily protein intake of 20 grams per 1,000 Calories, very similar to the figure (discussed earlier) of 40 grams of protein per day for the "average" adult, who needs about 2,400 Calories.

Growth of a human being, first as a fetus and then as an infant, is characterized at first by the formation of cells (cell proliferation) in all the organs of the body. Later, when the child grows up, growth is characterized by an increase in the mass of the cells and of the organs which they constitute. Thus, cell proliferation is normally followed by cell growth. Dietary protein is required for both these processes, but protein malnutrition seems to affect cell proliferation much more than cell growth. If protein malnutrition occurs at an early age, cell proliferation is slowed down, and the organs will never have their full complement of cells or reach their normal size, even if the diet is greatly improved later in the life of the child.

In the human brain, cell proliferation and cell growth occur very early in life, and are most rapid in the last few months of pregnancy and the first year after birth. Cell proliferation in the brain normally stops when the baby is six months old, and by age three the brain has already reached 80 percent of its adult weight. At that time the child has only reached 20 percent of its adult body weight. Thus the last months as a fetus and the first years of life are crucial to the development of the brain. Protein malnutrition during this period results in a physically smaller brain as reflected by a reduced head circumference. An examination of the brains of children who died from protein malnutrition during the first year of their life showed that they had 15 to 20 percent fewer brain cells than the normal child. These observations confirmed earlier experiments showing that rats and other animals fed protein-deficient diets in early life had physically smaller brains containing fewer cells than normal. Other experiments show that such animals are also deficient in their learning capacity. Because it is impossible to do controlled feeding experiments with children, it has been difficult to show conclusively that this is also the case in humans. Malnourished children, and children who have physically recovered from malnutrition, generally score lower on intelligence and adaptive-behavior tests than their counterparts who are adequately nourished and live in a similar environment. These studies suggest that protein malnutrition of infants (especially during the first year) may permanently restrict their mental abilities. This has frightening implications for the poor countries, where 500 million children are now growing up with physical and mental characteristics which may be inadequate to meet the challenges which will face them as adults.

VITAMINS, MINERALS, AND WATER

Vitamins

Vitamins are small molecules which are needed in the human diet in very small amounts. Whereas daily protein requirements are measured in grams, vitamin requirements are generally measured in milligrams or mg (thousandths of a gram). They are relatively small molecules, comparable in size to amino acids or sugars. But even in trace amounts they play important roles in the body. Most vitamins are *coenzymes*, molecules essential to make an enzyme do its work. For example, vitamin C is needed for the enzymatic formation of collagen, a substance important in wound healing and in the stability of the joints. Vitamin A is required in the biosynthesis of one of the pigments in the eyes. Vitamins are present in the food we eat, and are taken up in the body dissolved either in water (vitamins B and C) or in fats (vitamins A, D, E, K).

Although all living organisms contain nearly all the vitamins, some are particularly rich in certain vitamins and so are especially valuable food sources. Vitamin C is abundant in citrus fruits and is found in fresh vegetables. The B vitamins are most abundant in meats, wheat germ, and yeast. Cod-liver oil is a good source for the lipid-soluble vitamins A and D. Vitamin A is also found in yellow vegetables (squash, carrots, sweet potatoes), but vitamin D is not abundant in plants. Because many people are either unable or sometimes unwilling to eat the variety of foods necessary to get all the necessary vitamins, efforts have been made in some countries to add purified or manufactured vitamins to available foods. This process of fortification has been especially successful in the addition of vitamin D to milk.

Diets low in certain vitamins cause specific deficiency diseases. Lack of vitamin B_1 (thiamine) results in beriberi, a disease characterized by weak muscles and paralysis. Beriberi became much more common in Asia when mills started polishing the rice. This process removes the thiamine-rich outer layers of the grain. In those areas where polished rice is an important staple food, beriberi is still a very common vitamin-deficiency disease. At one time beriberi also occurred among people living in isolated villages in northeastern Canada, because bread made from white flour was their principal source of food during the long winter months.

A diet deficient in nicotinamide (also called niacin) causes pellagra, a disease characterized by skin lesions, diarrhea, and mental apathy. Nicotinamide can be taken up by the body, or it can be made from the amino acid tryptophan when other vitamins are present. Pellagra is a common disease among people who rely heavily on corn as their staple food. As was pointed out earlier (see Table 2.2), corn protein contains very little tryptophan. The large amount of leucine present in corn protein furthermore seems to prevent the conversion of tryptophan to nicotinamide.

A deficiency of vitamin D in the diet causes rickets, a disease characterized by weak and misshappen bones. Once very common, the incidence of this disease has been reduced greatly in the U.S. by vitamin D fortification of milk. Vitamin D increases the absorption of calcium from the intestinal tract and lowers the rate of phosphate excretion in the urine. As a result it raises the levels of phosphate and calcium in the blood and causes them to be deposited in the bones.

There is some controversy about whether the doses of vitamin intake recommended by nutritionists are too low. Some recent evidence indicates that large doses of vitamins may improve health in addition to preventing deficiency diseases. For example, 60 milligrams of vitamin C a day prevents the deficiency disease scurvy; but, according to Nobel prizewinner Linus Pauling, 2,000 milligrams a day (2 grams) decreases the incidence and shortens the duration of colds. Scientists now realize that much more research needs to be done to understand the role which vitamins play in human nutrition and health. Diets which are too *high* in certain vitamins can also result in physiological disorders.

Minerals

A growing number of minerals have been found to be essential for human life. Some minerals, such as calcium and phosphorus, are required in large amounts; others, such as iron or magnesium, are needed in smaller amounts; still others, such as copper, cobalt, or molybdenum, are required in trace amounts. Since many of these minerals are quite common in the liquids we drink and the foods we eat, nutritionists pay little attention to them. The minerals which cause special concern are those known to be deficient in certain diets. These are calcium, phosphate, iron, and iodine.

Large amounts of calcium and phosphate are needed for bone formation, but the body requires vitamin D in order to incorporate these minerals into bones. The Food and Nutrition Board of the U.S. government recommends an intake of 0.8 to 1.3 grams per day of each of these two minerals. Milk and milk products contain abundant amounts of both calcium and phosphate, which are also found in grain products, meat, and a variety of vegetables. In spite of this, many people do not ingest adequate amounts of calcium. A nutritional survey of the U.S. made in 1965 revealed that 30 percent of the persons surveyed had a calcium intake below the recommended allowance. Urban households on low incomes tended to have the most calcium-deficient diets.

Iron deficiency leads to anemia, a disease characterized by a general weakening of the body because there are not enough red blood cells. The red blood cells carry oxygen from the lungs to all the tissues, where the oxygen is used in the biochemical reactions which provide energy. Oxygen is actually carried by the red, iron-containing protein, hemoglobin. When iron is lacking in the diet, the body cannot synthesize hemoglobin. Anemia is very prevalent among women, who need more iron than men because of the loss of blood (and hence iron) during menstruation. The recommended daily intake of iron is 18 mg for women and 10 mg for men. Normal diets provide between 10 and 15 mg of iron per day, which is not enough for those women who lose a substantial amount of blood during menstruation.

The iron requirements of pregnant women are very high, and anemia is especially prevalent among them. One-third of all mothers' deaths at childbirth result from iron-deficiency anemia. A newborn child contains about 400 mg of iron; and the growth of the placenta, and the loss of blood during delivery, use up about another 300 mg. The total iron requirement for a pregnancy is therefore about 700 mg, or 2.5 mg per day, *in addition* to the basic metabolic requirement for iron. Since only 10 percent of the dietary iron is normally absorbed by the body, the diet should contain an extra 25 mg per day, for a total of 40 to 45 mg per day. This high need for iron can usually only be satisfied by iron supplements.

Although the body needs only small amounts of iodine (about 0.1 mg per day), the World Health Organization estimates that as many as 200 million people suffer from goiter, a disease caused by iodine deficiency. Goiter is characterized by an enlarged thyroid gland, a sluggish metabolism, a tendency to obesity, and an enlargement of the face and neck. The iodine content of many foodstuffs is variable, and in many areas of the world it is so low that a normal diet does not provide the body with enough iodine. Iodine deficiency can be most easily prevented by the fortification of table salt with iodide.

Water

We take water so much for granted that we often do not realize how critical it is for life. The water content of the human body is very high, and varies from 70 percent in a lean person to 50 percent in an obese person.

The importance of water as a foodstuff was demonstrated when it was shown that animals on a starvation diet still survived after losing all their stored fats and carbohydrates and about half their protein. However, a loss of 10 percent of their water was very serious, and a loss of 20 percent usually resulted in death. Water must be taken in continuously to prevent the body from dehydrating and to maintain the proper balance of salts in body fluids. Water plays several important roles in the body. It is, first of all, the medium in which all biochemical transformation of the other nutrients takes place. Water helps to carry nutrients from the gastrointestinal tract into the bloodstream, because the nutrients are dissolved in water. Water is also important in excretion; waste products are dissolved in it and excreted as urine. Water helps regulate body temperature by absorbing the heat released by the respiratory activity of all the tissues; much of the heat is used to transform liquid water into water vapor during the process of perspiration. An average person (60 to 70 kg) needs to take in 1,800 to 2,500 grams of water each day. About half of this is excreted as urine, and the other half leaves the body as perspiration or in the expired air. Half a person's water intake comes from beverages; the rest is contained in food (some foods, such as fruits, contain up to 80 percent water).

CHAPTER 3

Plants as a Source of Food

PLANTS ARE HUMANITY'S MAJOR FOOD SOURCE

To remain in good health, people must eat both energy-producing foods (carbohydrates and fats) and a proper balance of the other nutrients (proteins, vitamins, minerals, and water). Nutritionists have long maintained that, in order to have this kind of healthy diet, people should daily eat foods from the four "basic food groups." The division of foods into these four groups, as shown in Figure 3.1, provides a useful guide for the people of the industrialized countries, where food is abundant. It is, however, a recipe for the rich, because it relies heavily on animal products. Most people in the world cannot afford the luxury of selecting a daily diet that contains both dairy and meat products. Instead, they rely heavily on plant products as their source of food. This fact can easily be illustrated by comparing the food sources of calories and proteins in the diets of Americans and Indians (see Table 3.1). Not only is there a difference in the total amount of food available to and consumed by the average person in the two countries, but Indians get a much greater proportion of their calories and proteins from plant products. They eat only small amounts of meat, eggs, poultry, milk, and milk products.

Plants Provide Most Human Calories and Protein

In examining where the human population gets its food, nutritionists and agricultural economists are concerned primarily with calories and proteins. If a diet contains enough of these components, it will usually contain enough vitamins and minerals. On a global scale (see Table 3.2), plants directly provide 88 percent of the calories (carbohydrates and fats) and

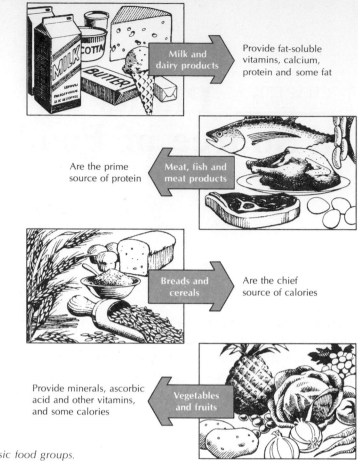

Provide fat-soluble vitamins, calcium, protein and some fat

Milk and dairy products

Meat, fish and meat products

Are the prime source of protein

Breads and cereals

Are the chief source of calories

Provide minerals, ascorbic acid and other vitamins, and some calories

Vegetables and fruits

FIGURE 3.1.
The four basic food groups.

Table 3.1. Sources of protein and calories in the food supplies of India and the U.S.A.[a]

Foodstuff	Source of calories		Source of protein	
	India	U.S.A.	India	U.S.A.
Cereals and starchy foods	71%[b]	23%	66%	20%
Sugars	9	17	—	—
Protein-rich seeds (e.g. beans, lentils)	9	3	20	2
Fruits and vegetables	1	5	1	4
Fats and oils	4	17	—	—
Milk and milk products	5	11	9	24
Meat, poultry, egg, and fish	less than 0.5	24	2	48

[a]Data from R. Revelle, "Food and Population," *Scientific American,* Sept. 1975, pp. 161–170.
[b]Read as "71 percent of all calories consumed in India are derived from cereals and starchy foods," and similarly for the other entries.

Table 3.2. Dietary calories and protein
for the human population.[a]

Region	Percent of calories from plant foods	Percent of protein from plant foods
World	88	80
Asia	95	78
Africa	93	79
Europe	81	53
Latin America	85	76
Oceania	65	30
North America	68	30

[a]From U.S. Department of Agriculture.

80 percent of the protein that human beings consume; the rest comes from animal products. As Table 3.2 shows, although the relative contribution of plants and animals to energy and protein intake varies from region to region, human beings are overwhelmingly dependent on plants as a source of energy and protein. Many different plant products are used for food in different parts of the world, but often the population in one area relies heavily on only one plant, the staple food, for most of its calories.

By far the most important staples are the cereals wheat and rice. Annual production of each is now around 350 million metric tons; more than ⅓ of the cultivated land is used to produce these two crops. Wheat is the dominant staple in 43 countries located in North America, Europe, North Africa, and the Near East, and rice is the dominant staple in most of Asia, an area which contains more than half the world's population. The world production of corn is nearly as large as that of wheat or rice, but corn supplies only about 5 percent of humanity's calories, because most of the corn is used as animal feed. Corn, which once was the dominant staple throughout the Americas, now occupies that position only in most of Central and South America. Root crops (white potatoes, sweet potatoes, yams, and cassava) supply humanity with 7 percent of its needed calories. White potatoes are grown primarily in Europe, and although they are an important source of calories, especially in Eastern Europe, they are not the dominant staple in any particular country. Sweet potatoes are the dominant staple in Nigeria and Ghana, and cassava (manioc) is the dominant staple in a few countries in Africa and Latin America. Although root crops supply not nearly as much energy to humanity as either wheat or rice (7 percent as against 20 percent), their annual production far exceeds that of wheat or rice. Annual production of root crops is around 550 million tons. Most grains contain at least 70 percent starch, whereas root crops contain only 25 percent starch or other carbohydrates. Thus it takes three tons of root crops to supply the same amount of energy as one ton of cereal grain. However, root crops have a much greater calorie productivity per unit land area than cereals; a hectare of potatoes yields 2 to 2.5 times as many calories as a hectare of wheat or rice.

The seed staples, have, generally speaking, a favorable protein content (8 to 15 percent of the dry weight); whereas the roots and tubers have a much lower protein content (1 to 3 percent). The ratio between protein and carbohydrates is often expressed as grams of protein per 100 Calories (see Figure 3.2). We saw earlier that an average adult should have a daily food intake of 40 to 60 grams of protein and 2,500 to 3,000 Calories, or about 2 grams of protein per 100 Calories. Staples which contain two or more grams of protein per 100 Calories are therefore also good sources of protein. This is reflected by the figures in Table 3.3, showing where the world population gets its dietary protein. More than half of it (55 percent) comes from the seed staples wheat, rice, and corn; another 13 percent is provided by the protein-rich seeds of legumes (peas, chickpeas, beans, lentils, cowpeas). The roots and tubers provide only 7 percent of the total. Animal products supply 20 percent of human beings' dietary protein, but most of this is consumed in the industrialized countries of the western world.

The areas of the world which rely heavily on plants as their source of protein (see Table 3.2) are generally those where hunger is prevalent (see Figure 2.4). Why should this be so? Thousands of healthy vegetarians can attest to the fact that animal products are not necessary for good health. The relationship between source of dietary protein and hunger is complex, but basically it results from the fact that these same countries, which have high rates of population increase, have not been able to increase their food production enough to even keep up with the increase in population. The lower protein-to-energy ratio of plant foods in comparison with animal foods (Figure 3.2) and the low protein score of plant proteins when compared with animal proteins (Table 2.2) also help explain the correlation between hunger and dependence on plant protein. Plant proteins are usually low in certain essential amino acids, and heavy reliance on a single staple often provides an inadequate supply of these. This deficiency can be corrected by supplementing the diet with plant proteins from different sources

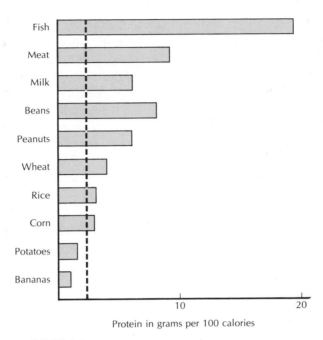

FIGURE 3.2.
Protein-calorie ratios of several foods. The dashed line shows the approximate adult daily dietary requirement for protein. (Data from F.A.O.)

(e.g., by mixing cereals and legumes) or by including small amounts of animal proteins in the diet. Unfortunately, these alternatives are not available to many people, and as a result protein malnutrition is widespread.

Conversion of Plant Protein to Animal Protein

If animal proteins have a higher nutritional value for human beings than plant proteins because they have a higher protein score, why not convert more plant protein into animal protein by raising more livestock and producing more milk and cheese? In the past, production of animal products depended entirely on food sources that human beings cannot eat anyway. Herbivores, such as cattle, sheep, and goats, can live entirely on grass and other plants which human beings cannot easily digest. Pigs and poultry can live in the farmyard or in the woods, where they find insects, seeds, and kitchen scraps. In many areas of the world, pigs still perform the essential service of converting garbage into meat. The fish and shellfish which human beings eat depend on the phytoplankton in the sea (either directly or indirectly) as their source of food. When animal protein is produced in this way, it comes to people "cheaply," because food sources of little value to human beings are converted into valuable foodstuffs.

In recent years, the production of animal protein has come to depend increasingly on food sources which human beings could eat themselves. Human beings and their domesticated animals are competing for the same food. Modern animal husbandry uses feedlots and factory farms, where the composition of the animal feed is constantly monitored in order to achieve spectacular results, such as chickens which lay an egg nearly every day of the year, dairy cows which produce 1,500 liters of milk a year, and sows which produce litters of 15 piglets which, six months later, together weigh 2,000 kg. This intensive production depends heavily on the use of wheat, corn, skim milk, soybeans, fish-protein concentrate, and other foods which human beings could consume directly. The feeding of these animals has also become extremely sophisticated. Computers are used to calculate the cheapest and best mixtures of foodstuffs, taking into account the composition, protein score, and price of each one, and the requirements of the animals. Synthetic amino acids (especially methionine) are now widely used to adjust the protein score when necessary. Millions of infants are suffering from protein malnutrition while the cattle in modern feedlots munch their scientifically controlled rations.

This use of grain and other high-quality foods to produce animal protein would be advantageous on a global scale if the conversion from plant to animal were efficient. Unfortunately, it is not. Like human beings, the animals use most of their food intake to support their own metabolism. While they are growing, they excrete a considerable quantity of the protein they consume. The efficiency of protein conversion from feedstuff to meat protein varies from a low of 5 or 10 percent (for herbivorous animals grazing on the open range) to a high of 30 or 40 percent (for production of eggs, broiler chickens, and milk). Recent increases in the prices of corn and soybeans have made meat and animal products an economic luxury, and an ecological luxury, that few people in the world can afford. Humanity's lot is obviously with plants as a source of food.

Plants as an Exclusive Source of Food

Eating meat every day is so culturally ingrained in technologically developed countries that it is easy to forget that many vegetarians never eat any meat at all. Some do it out of choice; some because of poverty. Some vegetarians do not exclude all animal products from their diets: many drink milk and eat milk products, and others include eggs in their diet.

Can we eat only plants and plant products and still remain in good health? The answer to this question depends on the meaning of the word "plants." The answer is "no" if we eat the familiar higher plants only, but "yes" if we include microbes such as yeast or bacteria. Neither plants nor animals can synthesize vitamin B_{12}; only microbes can. Meat is a good source of vitamin B_{12} because of the microbes living among the meat fibers, but most plants are a poor source. In India vegetarians eat seaweeds, the slime of which may be rich in B_{12}; some African tribes eat soil, in which there are abundant B_{12}-rich microbes; still others, religious sects in Asia, eat neither of these but still seem to survive, possibly because they have microbes that produce B_{12} living in their digestive systems. In most regions of the world, however, people on a strict vegetarian diet should supplement it with yeast or vitamin B_{12}. A deficiency of this vitamin results in a variety of diseases, usually culminating with degeneration of the spinal cord.

Plant proteins have low protein scores because they are low in certain essential amino acids. By carefully selecting a variety of plant proteins vegetarians can obtain a diet with a high protein score, for example, by combining cereals and legumes, as already mentioned. Some examples of how mixing staples affects the protein score are given in Table 3.3. Combinations of proteins should be eaten at the same meal, because the body cannot store amino acids. Careful planning is essential if one wants to derive an

Table 3.3. Protein score and protein content of various mixtures of staples.[a]

Cereal	Supplement[b]	Percent of Protein	Protein score
Wheat	None	11.2	62
	Groundnut	14.2	67
	Soybean	13.8	76
Corn	None	9.5	49
	Groundnut	12.6	58
	Soybean	12.2	67
Rice	None	6.7	69
	Groundnut	10.0	73
	Soybean	9.6	77

[a]From G. R. Jansen, "Amino-acid fortification of cereals," in A. Altschul, ed.; *New Protein Foods* (Academic Press, 1974), pp. 94–99.
[b]Adding 8 grams of protein concentrate to 100 grams of the staple.

adequate supply of protein from a vegetarian diet. It is far easier to ensure a proper diet by eating a *small* amount of animal protein to supplement a larger amount of plant protein. The large amounts of animal protein now consumed by most people in technologically advanced countries are nutritionally superfluous and are a drain on the global reserves of staple foods.

PLANT STRUCTURE AND HUMAN NUTRITION

Everyone who is at all concerned with the nutritional value of food knows that potatoes are more fattening per unit weight than celery, that wheat germ is more nutritious than lettuce, and that whole-wheat bread is better than sweet potatoes. The various parts of different plants contain very different amounts of nutrients. Some seeds are good sources of starch; others, of proteins; and still others, of fats. Leaves and stalks are poor sources of these three nutrients, but are rich in some vitamins, minerals, and roughage. Fruits are generally good vitamin and mineral sources, and storage roots and stems are rich in starch. The nutritional values of these plant organs largely depends on the roles they play in plant function. A better understanding of this dependence requires a discussion of the structure of the plant and of how it develops from a single cell to a fully mature organism capable of sexual reproduction.

Organs, Tissues, and Cells

Most plants are composed of two basic parts: the root system and the shoot system. The root system grows into the soil; its functions are to anchor the plant, and to take up minerals and water from the soil and transport them to the shoot system. The shoot system, which consists of stems and leaves, has two main functions: photosynthesis and the formation of reproductive organs (flowers). Each organ of the plant (stems, flowers, leaves, roots) is made up of various specialized tissues that perform specific functions, and each tissue contains one or more types of cells. The cells are the basic building blocks of the organism. A period of cell proliferation normally precedes a period of cell expansion in the formation of an organ, in plants as in humans. The formation of a new leaf starts with a period of cell division, during which nearly all the cells of the leaf are formed. The cells of the embryonic leaf then rapidly expand in size to form a mature leaf. At the same time, groups of cells become specialized to perform certain functions. In the leaf, for example, some cells are highly active in photosynthesis, whereas other cells are involved in support, and still others in protecting the leaf against dehydration.

The problem of wear and tear of the organ is solved entirely differently by plants and by animals. Animals continually replace the cells that have become ineffective. Plants cannot do this, but can continually make new organs. Indeed, plants have specific regions, called *meristems*, whose function is to continually produce new cells (meristematic cells), new tissues, and new organs. Every cell in a plant—and there are usually millions of cells—was derived from a dividing meristematic cell. When, after division, the different cell types take on specialized structures and specialized functions, they still retain many of their original features. As a result, different cell types have many common features, as well as those which distinguish them.

Meristematic cells, like all plant cells, are surrounded by a rigid *cell wall* (see Figure 3.3). This structure consists largely of carbohydrates, the most abundant being the undigestible (by humans) cellulose. This wall

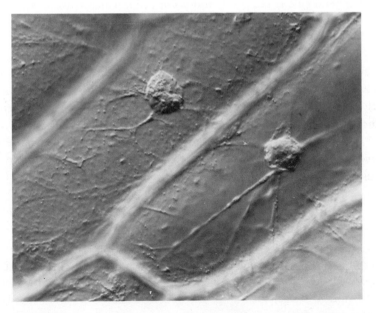

FIGURE 3.3.
Photograph of a meristematic cell. (Photo courtesy of Dr. M. McCully.)

encloses the living substance of the cell, *protoplasm*. Protoplasm is over 80 percent water; but the remaining 20 percent contains the chemicals necessary for life and useful for human nutrition. Protoplasm is rich in proteins and many vitamins. The microscope reveals several structures in protoplasm. Among these are the *cell membrane*, which controls the flow of chemicals in and out of the cell, and the prominent *nucleus*, which controls cell function. A third important structure in the plant cell is the *vacuole* which stores wastes and products not needed by the cell. It has nutritional value for human beings because it contains both vitamins and minerals.

Plant Cell Types

Meristematic cells occur only in meristems, tissues which specialize in cell division. They are small cells which are rich in protoplasm, have a thin cell wall, and contain several small vacuoles. In terms of percentage by weight, meristems contain a large amount of protoplasm, and they have a high nutritional value for human beings. However, meristematic cells usually constitute only a small fraction of the total plant. The only exception to this general rule is the plant embryo or *germ*, which consists almost entirely of meristematic cells and has a high nutritional value.

Parenchyma cells are much larger than meristematic cells, with somewhat thicker cell walls, and more protoplasm. Most of the cell volume is taken up by a large central vacuole, so that the protoplasm lies in a thin layer between the cell wall and vacuole. Parenchyma cells are normally found in leaves, young stems, and fruits, where they carry out many of the vital functions of the plant, such as photosynthesis. In terms of percentage by weight, such plant organs are poor in protein (protoplasm) and rich in cellulose (cell wall), vitamins, and minerals (vacuole).

Food storage cells in plants resemble parenchyma cells in their large size and small amount of protoplasm. The cell volume is not taken up by a large vacuole, but by many food-storage bodies, which contain either protein, fat, or starch and sometimes minerals. Such cells are normally abundant in seeds, in storage roots, such as sweet potatoes, and in subterranean storage stems, such as potato tubers. Plants store these foodstuffs in order to use them later. Some plants store mostly starch (potatoes, cereal grains); others also store large amounts of protein (seeds of leguminous plants, such as peas, beans, and lentils); and still others store mostly fat (peanuts, coconut). Food-storage cells, therefore, are the most important plant-cell types for human nutrition.

Conductive tissue cells function in the transport of a variety of substances from one plant part to another. For example, water and minerals flow from the roots to the leaves; sugar is transported from the leaves to the roots; plant hormones are transported within the plant in all directions. This conduction occurs in the specialized cells of the plant transport system. These cells have very thick cell walls and some of them have no protoplasm or vacuole. Such cells obviously have no nutritional value for humans, since they consist entirely of cellulose and other nondigestible cell-wall substances, but they contribute to human health by providing roughage. Conductive tissues are found in all the plant organs, but especially in the roots and stems. They contribute only a small proportion of the total tissue when these organs are young; whereas older stems, such as tree trunks, consist almost entirely of conductive tissues. In tree trunks most of this conductive tissue is in-active, only the peripheral tissues—the inside of the bark and the outside of the wood—being alive and active.

SEEDS

The Formation of Seeds

Development in organisms which reproduce sexually, whether plant or animal, begins with a single fertilized egg cell. The egg and the sperm which unite in fertilization are normally produced in specialized reproductive organs. In plants, these organs are located in the flower. The female repro-ductive organs, carpels, contain a number of ovules, each of which has a single egg. The male organs, stamens, produce a large number of pollen grains, each containing two sperms. Flower structures vary from plant to plant species, but in general the flowers of the important cereal crops occur in clusters. In wheat (Figure 3.4) and rice, small flowers are connected to a central stalk termed a spike; here, both male and female reproductive organs are in the same flower. In corn, on the other hand, female flowers are in lateral ears and male flowers in terminal tassels, at different locations on the same plant.

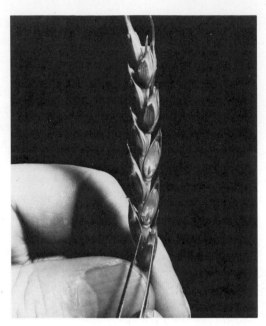

FIGURE 3.4.
A spike of wheat, with a flower exposed to show the reproductive organs. (Photo courtesy of U.S.D.A.)

The union of egg and sperm which initiates the development of a new plant occurs within the ovule. Depending on the species, pollen may come from the same plant (self-pollination, as in wheat) or from another plant of the same species (cross-pollination, as in corn). After fertilization, the cell that results from the union of egg and sperm undergoes many cell divisions and forms a multicellular embryo. Once the embryo is formed, food reserves (proteins, fats, carbohydrates, minerals) are deposited either within or next to the embryo. The developed embryo, the food-storage tissues and the hard outer seed coat together form the seed.

Seeds are usually formed during the active growing season. Once this season is over and the seeds drop to the ground, conditions for further growth of the parent plant are often unfavorable: winter or a dry season may arrive. If the plant is an annual, it will die; if it is a perennial, it will usually become dormant. In either case the seeds, which are the offspring of the plant, will survive the unfavorable growing period, because they are especially adapted to do so. Seeds have a very low water content (about 15 percent) and an unusually low metabolic rate. In this dry state they can survive for weeks, months, years, or even centuries, depending on the species and the environmental conditions. The seed allows a plant to survive until environmental conditions are suitable for growth. When conditions are favorable, the seed will germinate: the root and shoot of the embryo will start to grow. However, at this point the new plant does not yet have an autotrophic mode of nutrition: it cannot use the sun's energy, because it does not yet have any leaves. It obtains the energy, proteins, and minerals it needs by digesting the food in the storage tissues. Because the chemistry of this temporarily heterotrophic mode of nutrition strongly resembles that of animals, the food reserves stored in seeds (and other storage organs) are eminently suitable for use as human food. The food-storage tissues occupy most of the total volume of the seeds which figure prominently in human diets.

The formation of seeds represents an enormous biosynthetic effort for the plant, especially for the annual plants, which include most cereal grains and legumes, and which die once their seeds are produced. In annuals, photosynthesis occurs primarily in the younger green leaves, while the older leaves are already yellowing. When leaves yellow, not only does their green pigment, chlorophyll, disappear, but most of their proteins are broken down into amino acids. The amino acids from older leaves, newly synthesized amino acids, and sugars from the photosynthesizing young leaves are transported to the maturing seed, where they are used to make storage proteins and starch. Because plant seeds provide more than half the food of the human race, the biosynthesis of food reserves in the seed is one of the most important aspects of plant biochemistry.

Seed Dormancy

Once the seed is fully formed, it starts to lose water. This drying-out period is an important part of the maturation process of most seeds. Some plants have seeds which will germinate as soon as they have dried out. Many of our crop plants are in this category. However, the seeds of many plants of the temperate regions will not germinate immediately after ripening. After maturation, they become dormant, and this dormancy may last from a few weeks to several years. Such seeds will not germinate, no matter how suitable the environment, until dormancy disappears. In some species, the block against germination lies in the seed covering, which is impermeable to oxygen or water and which must be broken for development to occur. In other species, dormancy is governed by hormones. In still others, light seems to be involved in maintaining or breaking dormancy. Human populations generally select for crop-plant strains that do not exhibit dormancy, because a farmer usually wants seeds that will germinate immediately after sowing. Sometimes, however, dormancy of cereal grains is desirable, especially in regions where there is a great deal of moisture at harvest time. Dormancy will prevent the seeds from sprouting on the stalk before they are harvested.

The value of dormancy for the propagation of plants in natural conditions can be well-illustrated by looking at the role of dormancy in hazelnut germination. Hazelnuts must spend several months in a moist and cold environment before they will germinate. Normally, they are buried beneath the leaf-litter on the forest floor during the winter. This requirement for a cold period ensures that these seeds will not germinate in the fall of the same year that they are formed. Indeed, this would probably be an inappropriate time for germination, since the young seedlings might well be killed by frost. Some seeds may require more than a single winter of chilling, and the germination of seeds from a single crop will thereby be spread over at least two years. This spreading out creates a better chance that at least some of the seedlings will survive to become mature plants.

The Staff of Life

The cereal grains (wheat, rice, corn, rye, oats, barley, sorghum, and millets) can truly be called "the staff of life," for they are humanity's most important source of food. The domestication of cereals by human beings thousands of years ago marked the beginning of agriculture in Africa, Asia, and the Americas (see Chapter 6). Today, more than half the cultivated land on earth is used for growing cereals.

Botanically, cereals are grasses. They are usually annuals, or can be grown as annuals, and are efficient at gathering the sun's energy and transforming it into usable food. The fruit they produce is called a *grain*, a type of fruit which contains only a single seed surrounded by a thin, hard *fruit-wall*.* Cereal grains contain about 10 to 15 percent water, and as a result are eminently suited for long-term storage and long-distance transport. Well-filled granaries have been a sign of security and wealth throughout the ages.

The cereals used by the human race are adapted to a wide variety of soil and climatic conditions. *Rice* is grown primarily in Asia, in tropical

---

*A wheat "seed" or corn "seed" is actually a fruit, because it consists of a single seed surrounded by the fruitwall.

regions with abundant rainfall. Most of the rice is grown in submerged fields (paddies) in the plains adjacent to the big rivers of Asia. The fields are surrounded by dikes, and can be irrigated and drained when necessary. Plant physiologists have discovered that rice has an unusual physiology which allows it to grow submerged in water, a condition which kills most other plants. There are also various forms of upland rice which are cultivated in the same way as other seed crops. Upland rice has a lower yield, and its economic importance is not nearly as great as that of paddy rice.

Wheat is grown primarily in areas which are too dry and too cold for either rice or corn. Wheat grows best where the climate provides cool weather and moisture in the spring, followed by a sunny summer with a dry period at harvesting time. This weather pattern is found in parts of North America, in large parts of Europe, including the U.S.S.R. and in China. The leading producers of wheat are the U.S.S.R., the U.S.A., China, Canada, France, and India.

Wheats can be grouped in two categories: winter wheat and spring wheat. These names are derived from their planting times in the Northern hemisphere. In the Northern hemisphere, winter wheat is planted in the fall at the end of the growing season; the young plants become dormant during the winter. In the spring they start to grow again, and the crop is ready for harvest in early summer. Spring wheat, on the other hand, is planted in the spring, and it produces a crop during the same growing season.

Corn (also called maize outside the U.S.A. and Canada) grows best in areas that have a long growing season with hot summers and that receive abundant rainfall. Corn can be grown in many parts of the world, but other cereals are often preferred for cultural reasons. The world production of corn equals that of wheat and rice, and much of it is used as animal feed. The U.S.A. produces nearly half the world's crop, but 90 percent of it is used to fatten cattle and pigs.

Rye is grown primarily in Europe. It grows well in cool, dry areas, and can be successfully cultivated on soils which are too poor for growing other grains—as can *barley*, most of which is used for animal feed or for making beer. The world production of *oats* has been declining since tractors began replacing horses. Oats are grown primarily in North America and Europe. They are used for animal feed and to make a variety of breakfast cereals.

Sorghum grain is an important food source in Africa and Asia. The U.S.A. is the world's leading producer of sorghum, most of which is used as cattle feed. Sorghum, like corn, requires a hot summer, but it can be grown in areas with less rainfall and on much poorer soils. The recent discovery of a lysine-rich strain of sorghum may well increase its potential as a human food source.

Several different grain-producing plants are classified as *millets*. They grow in hot, dry areas, and are used as food crops in Africa and Asia. The yields of millets are usually low, but a crop can be produced in a short time, on poor soils, and with primitive methods of cultivation.

Cereal grains contain 10 to 15 percent water, 8 to 14 percent protein, 70 to 75 percent carbohydrate, and 2 to 7 percent fat, as well as a variety of minerals and vitamins. These nutrients are not evenly distributed through-out the grain, but are concentrated in various structures (see Figure 3.5). The outer layers of the grain, which form a protective cover, are composed of dead cells, which have only indigestible cell walls and no protoplasm. Contrary to popular belief, these layers are not rich in vitamins or minerals. The embryo or germ consists of a small root and a small shoot. Its meriste-matic cells are rich in proteins, fats, several B vitamins, and vitamin E. They also are rich in sugar, which accounts for the sweet taste of wheat germ. The bulk of the seed is taken up by the food-storage tissue or *endosperm*. The outer layer of the endosperm, called the *aleurone layer*, consists of cells

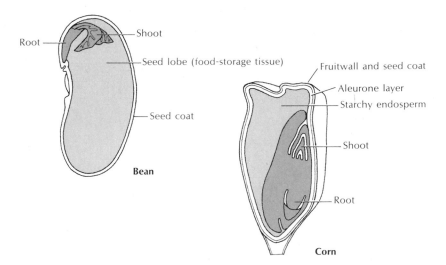

FIGURE 3.5.
Cross sections through a typical grain (corn) and a typical legume seed (bean).

which contain numerous protein bodies and are rich in nicotinic acid (niacin) and several important minerals (calcium, magnesium, phosphate, potassium). The central portion of the endosperm, called the starchy endosperm, consists of large cells tightly packed with starch granules embedded in a matrix of protein. The endosperm contains about 70 percent of the total protein, but the protein score of the endosperm proteins (the food-reserve proteins) is lower than that of the proteins in the embryo.

Throughout history, human beings have devised different ways of preparing cereal grains for eating. If the grains are eaten whole, they simply pass through the body; so humans have learned to pound, grind, parch, cook, roast, or soak the grains so that the body will be able to extract the nutrients more fully. In ancient times wheat was milled by simply pounding the grain in a mortar with a pestle or by shattering it between millstones. Today, the grain is squeezed first between steel rollers, then separated into its different parts: the bran (outer protective layers, aleurone, and some of the endosperm), the germ, and the endosperm. White flour and many break-fast cereals are made from the starchy endosperm, which is ground up into a powder. The polishing of rice also removes the protective covering struc-tures as well as the aleurone layer. Polished rice and white flour have the starch and proteins from the endosperm, but lack the vitamins (B and E), minerals, fat, and protein of the other parts.

Is white bread made out of bleached flour nutritious, or is it only a source of "empty" calories? Since ancient times, white bread has had greater social status than brown bread. Claims that brown bread is more nutritious than white have often been made: Greek and Roman writers described brown bread as symbolic of the simple life of country folk and better than the white bread of the rich. For a long time, brown bread meant not merely whole-wheat bread but bread containing flour from other plants (barley and legumes). Whole grain cereal, although not the ideal food, is a complete food, and milling it removes many essential nutrients. To circumvent this problem, white flour can be fortified with the missing nutrients. In the U.S., Canada, and Britain, riboflavin, nicotinamide, thiamine, and iron are re-introduced into white wheat flour, but the poor countries have not yet been able to undertake such large-scale fortification. The minerals of brown bread—calcium, magnesium, and phosphorus—are present in the aleurone, but in a chemical form unusable by humans, and only a small portion of these minerals is made available to humans by letting the bread dough rise for several hours. For this reason, wheat flour is fortified with calcium in

Great Britain. In addition, amino acids, such as lysine, can be added to improve the protein score of the flour. Such enrichment increases the protein score to 80 percent, far above that of whole-wheat flour. Lysine-enriched flour is now being used in Japan. Thus, the possibilities of fortification blur the nutritional distinction between brown and white bread.

Poor Man's Meat
The large protein-rich seeds of plants belonging to the family of the legumes—also called pulses—constitute one of mankind's important sources of food. Peas, kidney beans, lima beans, lentils, chickpeas, mungbeans, cowpeas, soybeans, peanuts, and broadbeans are the principal food legumes. In poor countries, the legumes are the most important high-protein food, and play the role that is played in the rich countries by meat and other animal products. Legumes are quite nutritious and contain 15 to 40 percent protein, 20 to 50 percent starch, and variable amounts of fat (from 2 to 3 percent in beans and peas to 50 percent in peanuts). They contain much more iron, five times as much riboflavin, and ten times as much thiamine as the same amount of cereals. As a result, legumes have become known as "poor man's meat." Although most legumes contain more protein than meat does, the nutritional score of their protein is much lower than that of meat proteins because they contain little methionine and tryptophan; soybean protein is the only exception to this general rule. The legume family also includes some plants which are used to make hay or silage for animals (clover, alfalfa, and various kinds of vetches), as well as a large number of trees.

Most plants are entirely dependent on the soil for their supply of nitrogen; legumes are not, because they can get much of their nitrogen from compounds that are produced by bacteria that live in their roots and use the nitrogen of the atmosphere. This direct use of atmospheric nitrogen is called nitrogen fixation. As a result of this process, such plants can grow on nitrogen-poor soils; they actually increase the nitrogen content of the soil. Leguminous plants can produce bumper crops without the benefit of synthetic nitrogen fertilizers.

It is unfortunate that a social stigma appears to be attached to the legumes. In the underdeveloped countries they are largely eaten by the rural poor and snubbed by city dwellers, even though the latter are very much in need of high-protein foods. The same situation often exists in the rich countries: in the U.S.A., beans are eaten primarily by the poor, and

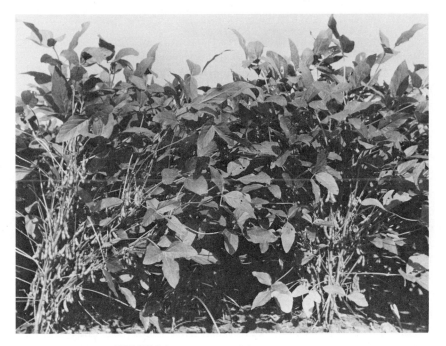

FIGURE 3.6.
Soybean plants. (Photo courtesy of U.S.D.A.)

few middle-class Americans would consider preparing a meal based on beans or lentils as the primary source of protein.

Soybeans are the most important legume, in terms of both the amount of protein they yield (35 to 40 percent) and their protein score (67 percent). Soybean production in the U.S. has increased substantially in the last 40 years, and the cash value of the annual crop now rivals that of wheat and corn. More than 20 million hectares, an area large enough to adequately feed all the inhabitants of New York, Chicago, Los Angeles, and Washington, D.C., are devoted to soybean production, but almost none of the crop is directly consumed by man. Much of the soybean crop is processed for oil, which is used to make shortening, margarine, and salad oil. The oil is extracted with solvents, and the protein-rich cake remaining after the extraction is used as animal feed. A small portion finds its way into food as flour (to increase the protein content of bread), as an ingredient in soups, or as a meat extender in various prepared products, such as hot dogs.

STEMS, LEAVES, AND ROOTS

Growth of the Plant

With the appearance of conditions that break dormancy and allow germination, the seed first restores its former water content and swells. This rehydration triggers the two main events of germination: embryo growth and use of the seed's food reserves. The embryo growth depends on use of the reserves, because it is not until green leaves have formed on the seedling that it can grow autotrophically. Its initial growth depends on the carbohydrates, fats, proteins, and minerals present in the storage tissues of the seed. The starch, fats, and proteins are first broken down into their simple-molecule constituents (sugar, fatty acids, and amino acids), and these are then absorbed and used by the growing embryo. Chemically, this is the same digestive process that takes place when people eat these seeds. It was recently shown that this digestive process is controlled in cereal grains by a hormone present in the embryo.

As the embryo absorbs the digested products of the seed's storage material, it uses them to build more cells and to expand cells once they are made. Within a few days, a recognizable root is growing down through the soil and the shoot (stem and leaves) is pushing above ground. Once the shoot is above ground, light causes the stem to elongate less rapidly and the leaves to expand. Soon, the green pigment chlorophyll appears, and the plant can begin to carry on photosynthesis and cease to be dependent on the seed reserves.

Even in a very young seedling, the three major organs that make up the mature plant—root, stem, and leaf—can be distinguished. The development and growth of these organs are complex, highly integrated processes. When plant growth is examined in terms of what the cells are doing, the development of these organs is seen to involve three basic processes: cell division, cell enlargement, and cell differentiation.

A good example of the sequence of these processes is found at the tip of the growing root. At the very tip, just behind the protective root cap, is a meristem, a region of continuously dividing cells (see Figure 3.7). These new cells then become from ten to a hundred times larger; behind the region of cell division there is thus a region of cell elongation. Finally, once they are fully enlarged, these cells specialize, depending on location, into the various cell types of the root; behind the enlargement region there is thus

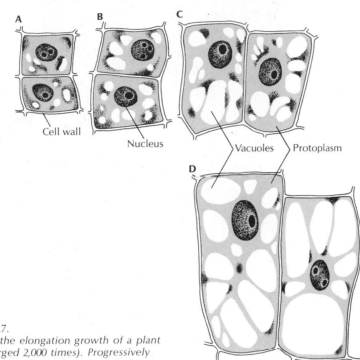

FIGURE 3.7.
Stages in the elongation growth of a plant cell (enlarged 2,000 times). Progressively older cells are shown from A to D.

a region of cell differentiation. This sequence is always maintained as the root grows through the soil.

Growth in length of the root is accompanied by the formation of lateral roots, which grow from the inner tissues of the main root. These lateral roots will in turn form more lateral roots, until the plant has established a widely branched root system capable of taking up water and minerals from a large volume of soils. An average four-month-old rye plant has about 700 miles of roots!

In addition to having an extensive root system, many plants greatly increase the area exposed to the soil by forming root hairs (see Figure 3.8). These are tiny projections from individual cells on the surface of the root. Most roots have billions of root hairs, which increase the root's absorptive surface area many times over. For an average four-month-old rye plant, this surface area is about 1,000 square meters—all for a three-foot-high plant. To provide the plant with water and mineral nutrients, the root system

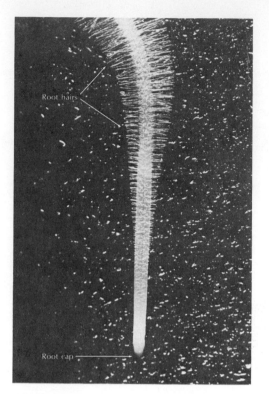

FIGURE 3.8.
Root hairs on a radish seedling. (Photo courtesy of Dr. M. McCully.)

must grow continuously; new roothairs are always being formed, as the older ones die off. Storage of food reserves is another important function of the root system. Some biennial plants, such as beets and carrots, develop a thick, fleshy taproot at the end of the first growing season. The reserves stored in this taproot are used at the beginning of the second growing season, when the plants flower and form seeds. Other plants develop numerous fleshy, tuberous roots for food storage and vegetative reproduction.

The processes involved in the growth of the shoot are generally similar to those for the root. A shoot consists of a stem and of leaves, which are attached to the stem at points called nodes. The stem portions between the nodes are the internodes (see Figure 3.9). The growing region of the stem is located at the tip within the terminal bud, which contains a meristem, a region of continuously dividing cells, which produces all the cells for the embryonic leaves and the internodes. Below the meristem lies a zone

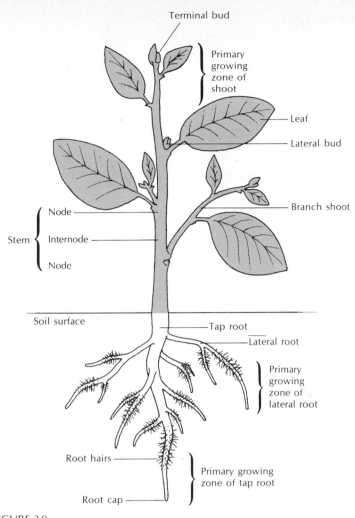

FIGURE 3.9.
Typical external features and mode of growth of the shoot and root systems.

of cell expansion, where these cells enlarge to their full size. While the cells are expanding, they are also differentiating into the different cell types of the shoot. Growth of the shoot in length is accompanied by the formation of side branches, which grow from quiescent buds on the side of the stem. Branching of stems is not a random process, but is controlled by a hormone that is produced in the bud at the top of the main stem. This hormone is *auxin,* which is transported downward and suppresses the growth of side branches. Side branches may form further down the stem, where the effect of the hormone is diminished. If the top bud is removed, the top will branch, and one of the new branches will become the main one and eventually suppress the growth of the others.

Root and shoot formation are not independent of each other. Indeed, in most plants there seems to be a constant ratio between the mass of roots and the mass of shoots. Cutting either one slows down the growth of the other. This balance may be controlled by hormones. In some plants, roots produce the hormone *cytokinin*, which is transported to the shoot and maintains growth. When cytokinin production in the roots slows down, the plant grows less vigorously and starts to yellow.

Vegetative Reproduction and Propagation

In addition to sexual reproduction, marked by flowering and seed formation, many plants can also reproduce asexually. In *asexual* or *vegetative reproduction*, new plants are formed, not from seeds, but from specialized structures of the root, stem, or leaf (the vegetative organs of the plant). In nature, such vegetative reproduction is often carried out by means of horizontal stems or roots, which allow the plant to spread over a larger area (see Figure 3.10). The strawberry is a familiar plant with this mode of

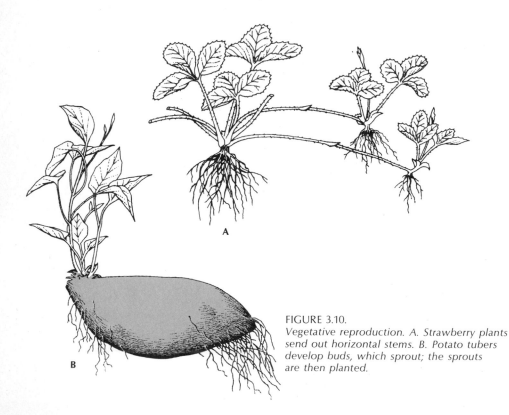

FIGURE 3.10.
Vegetative reproduction. A. Strawberry plants send out horizontal stems. B. Potato tubers develop buds, which sprout; the sprouts are then planted.

reproduction. It sends out *runners* (horizontal stems), which make new plants by sending down roots and forming leaf clusters at some of the places where they touch the ground. Horizontal stems which grow underground may become thick and fleshy and form *tubers*. Each tuber can give rise to a new plant when the parent plant has died. A potato plant propagates itself thus, by forming tubers (modified, underground stems) which will sprout the next spring. Many of the specialized structures involved in vegetative propagation are at the same time food storage organs and enable the plant to survive adverse conditions, as are the tuberous roots which in some plants (sweet potatoes, cassava) are a means of vegetative reproduction.

When people aid this process of vegetative reproduction, it is termed *vegetative propagation*. This method is used in the propagation of potatoes, sweet potatoes, berries, nuts, and a variety of fruit trees and ornamental plants. The advantage of asexual reproduction is that all the offspring have exactly the same characteristics as the parent plant. This is especially important when the parent is a genetic hybrid whose sexually produced offspring will not be the same as the parents. For example, an apple tree grown from a seed will not usually produce apples of the same quality as the parent plant. Vegetative propagation ensures a maintenance of high quality in these plants.

Plants which produce specialized structures for vegetative reproduction are easily propagated. Thus pieces of potato tubers or of the tuberous roots of the sweet potato will "sprout" and produce new plants when they are put in the soil. Other plants, such as sugarcane, pineapple, cassava, and many ornamental plants, are propagated by stem cuttings. In these species, pieces of stem produce roots spontaneously when placed in moist soil. The discovery that the plant hormone auxin promotes the rooting of stem cuttings in many species has recently enlarged the list of plants which can be propagated in this manner. Many stem cuttings that would not ordinarily produce roots will do so after the lower end of the stem is dipped in a solution of auxin.

Roots, Stems, and Leaves as Food Sources

"Root crops," which include a wide variety of plants, are an important source of food for mankind. They provide about 8 percent of human energy intake. Potatoes, yams, sweet potatoes, cassava, carrots, and beets are all classified as "root crops," because they are all fleshy, underground storage organs (even though not all of them are true roots). Root crops have a much higher water content than seeds do (70 to 80 percent as compared to 10 or 15 percent in seeds); so they are more difficult to preserve and transport. Their protein content and protein-to-calorie ratio are also low; so they are not adequate by themselves for human nutrition. Wherever these crops are used as staples, they must be supplemented with high-protein foods. The most important root crop is the potato (also called the Irish potato or white potato), which originated in the Andean highlands. It grows best in a climate where cool nights alternate with warm days during the period the tubers are being formed. Such conditions are found in large parts of Europe, which produces more than 75 percent of the world's potatoes.

Sweet potatoes and cassava (also called manioc) are two important tropical root crops, both of which probably originated in South America. The sweet potato has a higher nutritive value than the white potato, especially in vitamins A, B, and C and in calcium. China and Japan are the major producers and consumers of sweet potatoes.* Cassava plants adapt well to poor soils and casual cultivation, and are widely used in some of the shifting agricultural systems of the tropics. With little care, a cassava field may yield 15 tons of fresh roots per hectare. The roots contain very little protein and are about 30 percent starch. Sugar beets are another important root crop. They provide 35 percent of the world's sugar. Like potatoes, beets grow best in areas where warm days alternate with cool nights during the period when the sugar is being deposited in the storage root. As a result, their distribution is similar to that of the potato: Europe accounts for 80 percent of the sugar-beet production.

The stems and leaves of a wide variety of wild and domesticated plants are eaten as vegetables. They supply human beings primarily with minerals and certain vitamins (C and E). Different varieties of the cabbage family (e.g., head cabbage, cauliflower, broccoli, kale, collard greens) are mankind's most important leafy vegetables, and are rich in calcium and vitamin C. The amount of vitamin E in leafy vegetables increases with their "greenness"; dark green vegetables, such as collard greens, kale, or spinach, have much more vitamin E than iceberg head lettuce. The stem of a plant normally becomes stringier or woodier as it grows older, and only young stems are usually eaten. Asparagus, bamboo shoots, "chinese" bean sprouts, and palm shoots are only a few examples of young stems which are eaten in different

---

*Red-skinned sweet potatoes are mistakenly called "yams" in the U.S.; the true yams are the tubers of an entirely different tropical plant, of East Asian origin.

parts of the world. The economic importance of leaf and stem crops is difficult to estimate, because much of them are grown in small gardens by the consumers themselves.

The economically most important stem crop is sugar cane, which supplies 65 percent of the world's sugar. Sugar cane is a tropical grass which stores sucrose in its stalk. A highly successful plant-breeding program has created strains that have a high sugar content and that have greatly increased the yield of sugar. Sugar cane is mankind's most efficient crop, because it converts a larger proportion of the sun's energy into food than any other crop. Refined sugar, however, supplies man only with calories, and contains no other nutrients. The extraction of sugar from sugar cane involves crushing the stalks, squeezing out the juice, and boiling it to concentrate the sugar by removing the water. The remaining sticky liquid contains not only sugar but small amounts of proteins and minerals as well. If this liquid is dried, it yields a crude form of sugar which is considerably more nutritious than the refined sugar produced in modern sugar mills. This crude form of sugar is a dietary staple in Costa Rica and the Dominican Republic, where it supplies more than half the calories in the diet. Modern sugar refineries first remove the proteins and then allow the sugar to crystalize. The crystalized sugar is then separated from the dark-brown, mineral-rich sugary liquid (molasses), and further refined to yield a product free of all "impurities." Molasses is used as an animal feed or in the production of rum.

FLOWERS AND FRUITS

Sexual Reproduction

Sexual reproduction in a plant, as in most other organisms, requires the union of a sperm cell and an egg cell. The sperm and the egg cells are produced in specialized reproductive organs located in the flower. A flower consists of *sepals* (often green), *petals* (often vividly colored), male reproductive organs called *stamens,* and female reproductive organs called *carpels.* All these structures are modified leaves which originate in the flowerbud in the same way that normal leaves originate in a vegetative bud.

In many annual plants the formation of the flower involves the conversion of the terminal vegetative bud, which would ordinarily produce more shoot tissues, into one which produces a flower. Once the flowering signal has been received by the bud, the embryonic "leaves" develop into sepals, petals, stamens, and carpels instead of differentiating into leaves. The same signal also prevents the elongation of the internodes, so that all the parts of the flower appear to be attached at the same point on the stem.

In many plant species, the relative durations of day and night provide the plant with the signal to produce flowers (see Figure 3.11). Chrysanthemums normally flower in the fall. However, if mature plants are kept in a greenhouse under conditions which simulate the length of the summer day (16 hours of light and 8 hours of darkness), they will not flower no matter what the temperature or time of year is. If, on the other hand, the plants are kept under conditions which simulate winter (8 hours of light and 16 hours of darkness), they will flower even in summer! Plants which flower when the days are short are termed "short day plants" (chrysanthemums, rice); those that need long days are termed "long day plants" (oats, winter wheat). The upper leaves of the plant "sense" the photoperiod, for if they are removed, the plant will not flower even in the correct daylength. The suggestion has been made that the leaves receive the photoperiodic stimulus, then synthesize a "flowering hormone" and send it to the bud. Isolation of such a hormone would be of great practical importance, for with it one could

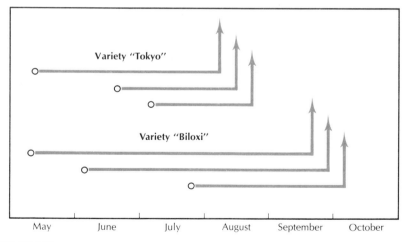

FIGURE 3.11.
Planting dates (0) and flowering dates (↑) of two varieties of soybeans. Despite the widely differing planting dates, all the plants flower close to the same time, because the flowering is triggered only by a certain length of day. (Data from the original research of W. Garner and H. Allard, "Effect of the Relative Length of Day and Night and Other Factors of the Environment on Growth and Reproduction in Plants," Journal of Agricultural Research, *18, 1920, 553–606.)*

induce flowering and seed formation at any time of year, and schedule harvests to suit the harvester, not the crops. Unfortunately, no one has yet isolated this hormone.

Because of photoperiodism, plants only flower in the proper season. This may be a disadvantage for the farmer, because he cannot grow more than one crop per year. Multiple cropping, which is practiced in many tropical areas where there is abundant water and sunshine, is only possible if the plants are insensitive to the photoperiod. The new strains of wheat and rice that form the basis of much of the recent increases in grain production in the underdeveloped countries have been selected to have exactly this property.

The fertilization of the egg cell by the sperm cell is followed by the growth of the embryo and the formation of the seed. Concomitant with seed formation, the wall of the ovary which surrounds the seed(s) is induced to form a fruit. The early development of the fruit (often called "fruit set") is dependent on hormones, especially auxin, produced by the growing embryo within the seed. These hormones stimulate the cells of the ovary to divide and form the fruit. Applications of auxin can induce flowers to develop into fruits without fertilization. The fruit acts as a vehicle for distributing the seeds of the plant. Some seeds are very light and are distributed by the wind (for example, those of maple or dandelion). Others may be distributed by water or animals. Most familiar to people are the edible fruits with their fleshy fruitwalls which must ripen to release their seeds. Ripening involves a number of changes which usually cause the fruitwall to soften while acids and starch are converted to sugar. The ripening process is controlled by the gaseous hormone ethylene, which is produced by the fruit. Commercial fruit companies can induce ripening at will by picking the fruits when they are "green," and then keeping them for a few days in chambers containing ethylene. This procedure has the advantage that the fruits can be handled and transported before they become soft as a result of natural ripening.

The formation of seeds and fruits often coincides with the advent of environmental conditions not suitable for growth. In annual and biennial plants, senescence and death accompany seed and fruit formation. Perennial plants may shed their leaves and become dormant. Leaf senescence is often signaled by the yellowing of the leaves, which is caused by loss of the pigment chlorophyll, and is accompanied by a rise in hormones which cause the terminal buds to become dormant and the leaves to drop off. Like flowering, the processes of senescence and dormancy are controlled by changes in daylength, and so represent a response of the plant to its environment.

Flowers and Fruits as Food

Most fleshy fruits are eaten raw, and are valued by people because they add variety and flavor to the diet, but they are relatively unimportant as a source of calories or protein. Some, such as the pineapple, are quite rich in sugar, and most are good sources of soluble vitamins and minerals. Citrus fruits and a variety of wild fruits are excellent sources of vitamin C. Other fruits, such as bananas, plantains, dates, coconuts, olives, avocadoes, mangoes, and breadfruit, supply considerable amounts of calories and protein.

Bananas and plantains (a related species, also called "mealy bananas") are rich in starch, and are important staples in several areas (Brazil, the Dominican Republic, and Central Africa). They have an unfavorable protein-to-calorie ratio and must be supplemented by protein-rich foods to ensure a proper diet. Latin America accounts for three quarters of the world's banana production, but most of these bananas are grown on large plantations and exported to the developed countries. In the tropical regions of Africa and Latin America, many houses have a few banana trees in their yards and the fruits from these trees contribute to the nutrition of the inhabitants of these areas.

The coconut is a very nutritious fruit because its white "meat" is actually the endosperm of the seed, and its nutritional value is greater than that of endosperm of cereal grains. Although coconuts are eaten extensively by the inhabitants of coastal tropical regions, most of the world's coconut production is diverted for the production of oil. The coconut "meat" is first dried in the sun, and oil is then squeezed out of the resulting product. The remaining press cake, which is rich in protein, is usually sold as animal feed.

Many other fruits and some flowers are also eaten as vegetables. Artichokes, broccoli, and cauliflower are fleshy flower heads, whereas tomatoes, peppers, okra, eggplant, cucumbers, and squash are fruits. These "vegetables" are similar to the leafy vegetables in that they supply human beings with minerals and vitamins.

CHAPTER 4

The Role of Energy in Crop Production

PHOTOSYNTHESIS

Green plants, being autotrophic organisms, can manufacture energy-rich organic substances by converting the radiant energy they receive from the sun into the chemical energy present in the bonds which link the atoms of organic molecules. This process of energy conversion, called photosynthesis, is of such key importance for food production that we will spend most of this chapter on a detailed discussion of photosynthesis and the factors affecting it.

Solar Radiation

The Earth receives from the Sun a constant stream of radiation in the form of visible light, infrared light (heat rays), radio waves, ultraviolet light, and x-rays. Most important of these for plant growth are the visible light and heat rays, which profoundly affect the rates at which plants can photosynthesize and grow. Radiation travels through space with a certain wave motion. Although all the solar radiation travels at the speed of light (about 186,000 miles per second), there is considerable variation in the length of the waves, that is, the number of wave motions per unit distance. Radiation with a shorter wavelength has more energy than radiation with a longer wavelength. Solar radiation of certain wavelengths is detected by our eyes as visible light of different colors. The shortest light waves stimulate in us the sensation of violet and the longest stimulate the sensation of red (see Figure 4.1). These light waves form the visible spectrum, and it is light in these wavelengths that plants use in photosynthesis. The visible spectrum, however, is only a small fraction of the range of wavelengths emitted by

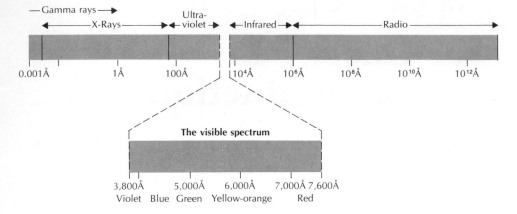

FIGURE 4.1.
A portion of the electromagnetic spectrum. Visible light constitutes a very small part of the total spectrum. Light of different visible wavelengths is perceived by humans as different colors. Wavelengths are in Ångstroms: 1 Ångstrom = 10⁻¹⁰ meter.

the Sun. For example, both shorter-wavelength (ultraviolet) and longer-wavelength (infrared) light reaches the Earth, although we cannot see them directly. The infrared radiation which impinges on the Earth provides it with heat.

The amount of solar radiation (light, heat, and other forms of radiation) which reaches a plant on the Earth's surface will vary according to the transparency of the atmosphere, the cloud cover, the position of the plant on the Earth (latitude), and the time of year. The angle at which sunlight hits the Earth has perhaps the most profound effect on the intensity of solar radiation. This angle is affected by the latitude and by the seasons. Figure 4.2 shows the amount of direct sunlight falling on a horizontal surface located outside the Earth's atmosphere. At the equator, seasonal variation is slight; whereas close to the poles (80° north latitude), incident light is zero in the winter and very high in midsummer. The annually changing temperatures in the midlatitudes and the polar regions, and the constant temperatures in the tropics, are a direct consequence of these radiation regimes. The Sun's rays strike the polar regions at a sharp angle, whereas they strike the equatorial regions almost perpendicularly. As a result, they must travel through more of the atmosphere before reaching the Earth in

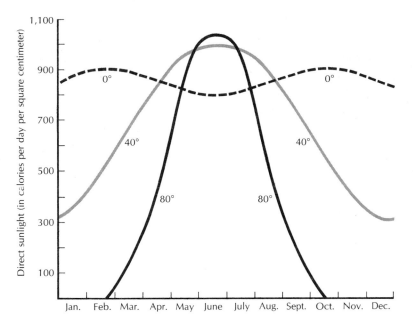

FIGURE 4.2.
Amount of direct sunlight hitting a horizontal surface at the upper atmosphere as a function of latitude and time of year. (From D. Gates, Man and His Environment: Climate, *Harper and Row, 1972, p. 28.)*

the polar regions, and there is more chance that the radiation will be scattered or absorbed before it reaches the Earth.

Another, and less obvious, factor which determines the temperature of the Earth is the reradiation of infrared rays back into the atmosphere. All this heat would be lost into space, except that the atmosphere acts like a pane of glass and reradiates most of the heat rays back to the Earth; this phenomenon is called the "greenhouse effect," and it has great impact on the global climate. Any significant alteration in the atmosphere could have drastic consequences: for example, an increase in the particulate matter and water vapor in the air could cause more of the infrared rays to be reradiated back to the Earth. Some meteorologists believe that this could raise temperatures on Earth enough to cause a partial melting of the polar ice caps and a rise in the water level of the oceans.

Photosynthesis

In 1771, Joseph Priestley performed an experiment which led to the current understanding of the importance of atmospheric gases in photosynthesis. He placed a mouse in a sealed jar, and observed that it died after a while. If, however, the mouse was put in a jar in which a candle had burnt, it died almost immediately, because, as Priestley put it, the candle had "exhausted" the air. In a third experiment, he put a twig from a mint plant in with the "exhausted" air; after a while, he added the mouse, and it did not die immediately. "Vegetation," he wrote, "restored the air. From these discoveries we are assured that no vegetable grows in vain but cleanses and purifies our atmosphere."

Chemists can now explain Priestley's experiment in terms of the exchange of gases between organisms and the atmosphere. The burning candle had "exhausted" the air of oxygen, and without a supply of this gas for respiration, the mouse died. The mint twig used the carbon dioxide remaining in the air to restore oxygen to the air by the process of photosynthesis, as shown in the following equation:

$$\text{Sunlight} + 6CO_2 + 6H_2O \rightarrow C_6H_{12}O_6 + 6O_2$$

$$\underset{\substack{\text{carbon} \\ \text{dioxide}}}{} \quad \underset{\text{water}}{} \quad \underset{\text{sugar}}{} \quad \underset{\text{oxygen}}{}$$

This equation does not show the great complexity of the process of photosnythesis, in which many biochemical reactions and intermediates are involved, but it does indicate that, in general, photosynthesis is the reverse of respiration as carried out by animals, plants, and most microorganisms. In respiration, oxygen combines with sugar to form carbon dioxide and water:

$$C_6H_{12}O_6 + 6O_2 \rightarrow 6H_2O + 6CO_2 + \text{energy}$$

A key difference between the two processes is in the "energy" term. Photosynthesis uses solar energy to link atoms together; respiration releases energy when the bonds between these atoms are broken again. This energy is released in a form which can be used to power all the energy-requiring reactions in an organism.

Photosynthesis occurs primarily in the leaves of green plants. A cross section of a typical leaf reveals that it is eminently suited to be a photosynthetic factory (see Figure 4.3). The leaf is thin and flat to maximize the surface area that receives sunlight. It contains "veins" of conductive tissue, so that water can be brought in and the sugar formed can be trans-

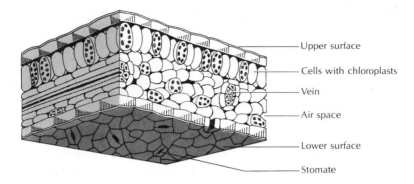

FIGURE 4.3.
A cross section through a typical leaf.

ported to other parts of the plant. The many air spaces between the cells facilitate gas exchange. In addition, the leaf surfaces, especially the lower one, are dotted with thousands of tiny pores, the stomates. These pores regulate gas exchange between the leaf and the atmosphere by their number and size. The plant can regulate the size of the stomates. For example, during the day, when sunlight is available, the stomates open and CO_2 enters the leaves. At night, when there is no light and photosynthesis does not occur, the stomates are closed. Finally, the cells nearest the upper surface of the leaf also contain many chloroplasts, the cellular structures which are the site of photosynthesis.

The light which falls on a leaf or any other object is either reflected from it, transmitted through it, or absorbed within it. Chloroplasts contain a pigment, chlorophyll, that absorbs light in the blue and red portions of the visible spectrum. The remaining wavelengths of sunlight are not absorbed by chlorophyll, and most are transmitted through the plant to the observer; so the leaf appears green. Once the chlorophyll has absorbed the radiant energy, it passes the energy to other molecules in the chloroplast. The energy, now in chemical form, is passed via a series of intermediates to the carbon atoms of carbon dioxide. These carbons are then linked to form glucose. The chlorophyll molecules, in the meantime, can now receive more light energy to replace what they passed along.

Once glucose is formed in the leaf, it can have a number of fates. Some of it is immediately converted to sucrose (see Figure 2.1B), and in this form it can be transported all over the plant. Most of it is converted to starch (see Figure 2.1C) and stored within the chloroplasts. The starch is usually digested again at a later time, and the resulting glucose can be used directly by the leaf cells or transformed into sucrose and transported all over the plant by the conductive tissues. The cells in different parts of the plant body use the products of photosynthesis for two different purposes: as a source of energy, and to build a great variety of complex organic molecules (e.g., cellulose, fats, proteins). Most cells in the interior of the plant body (stems, roots, flowers, seeds) are nonphotosynthetic, and the sucrose they obtain from the leaves is the only energy source they have. They may use this energy to carry out biochemical reactions, to take up minerals from the soil, or to transport substances. The products of photosynthesis are also used to make other molecules, if other necessary nutrients have been taken up from the soil. For example, by rearranging the carbon atoms of glucose and adding nitrogen in a suitable form, the plant can synthesize amino acids.

The Environment and Photosynthesis

The rate of plant growth is influenced by many environmental variables, such as the intensity of light, the temperature, the CO_2 concentration in the air, the amount of water of the soil, the O_2 concentration in the air, the alternation of night and day temperatures, and the length of the day. Many of these factors have a direct effect on the rate of photosynthesis; others affect the process of respiration.

The most obvious environmental factor that influences the rate of photosynthesis in a plant is the amount of light which hits the plant. Both the duration of the light period (number of hours of daylight) and the intensity of the light are important variables. The duration of the light period is simply the number of hours the plant can carry out photosynthesis. The intensity of the light affects the rate of the photosynthetic process. A plant with a certain number of chlorophyll molecules in its leaves can use a certain maximum amount of sunlight per second. If the light intensity is less than this maximum for a given plant, that plant will carry out photosynthesis more slowly than it could. For many crop plants there is a linear relationship between light intensity and photosynthetic rate (measured as the amount of CO_2 "fixed" per unit time into other molecules). The rise in CO_2 fixation with light intensity has its limit at the point where the plant's photosynthetic machinery is working at peak efficiency. Beyond this point, further increase in light intensity has no effect on photosynthesis. This light intensity required for maximal photosynthesis differs from species to species. In other words, as shown in Figure 4.4, corn can take much better advantage of high light intensities than orchard grass or maple can.

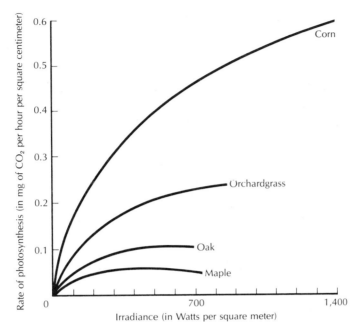

FIGURE 4.4.
The effect of light intensity on photosynthesis in four species.
(From J. Hesketh and D. Baker. Crop Science 7 (1967), 285–93, by
permission of the Crop Science Society of America.)

Another important factor in photosynthesis is the proportion of in-cident light actually intercepted by the leaves. If the plants are small (early in the season, in a field) or are sparsely placed, they will not intercept all the light. Photosynthesis in each plant may be maximal, but plant growth and crop production per unit area of land may be far from maximal. Agron-omists therefore select crop plants which are well-adapted to dense stands, so that the photosynthetic rate per unit area of land can be maximized. It has recently been demonstrated, for example, that corn plants whose leaves stand up straight intercept a greater proportion of the sunlight and produce higher yields than corn plants whose leaves droop down.

The concentration of carbon dioxide within the leaf, and the affinity of the photosynthetic enzymes for carbon dioxide, are other important variables that affect the rate of photosynthesis. The concentration of CO_2 in the leaf is limited by the concentration of this gas in the atmosphere (normally about 0.03 percent) and by its diffusion through the stomates into the leaf cells. At high light intensities, increases in CO_2 concentration up to 0.1 percent increase the rate of photosynthesis, because CO_2 can enter the leaf more rapidly. Higher concentrations of CO_2 (beyond 1 percent) are definitely poisonous to plants. In practice one can increase CO_2 concentration only in a closed chamber, such as a greenhouse. However, such experimentation has led to important conclusions on the key role of photosynthesis in crop production. Dr. R. W. F. Hardy and his coworkers of E. I. du Pont de Nemours and Company have experimented with soybean plants under different carbon dioxide concentrations to see if increases in photosynthesis also lead to increases in nitrogen in the seeds. Such an increase would be important for food production, since the nitrogen content of a seed indicates its protein content. Their results (see Table 4.1) show that doubling the CO_2 concentration led to a slight increase in the total weight of the plant body and its nitrogen content, but the weight and nitrogen content of seed pods was almost doubled. The nitrogen in the seeds was doubled because the nitrogen-fixing bacteria in the roots of the soybeans were able to synthesize much more atmospheric nitrogen into ammonium, which the plants used to make amino acids, and hence proteins. The experiment by Hardy and his colloborators implies that increasing the flow

Table 4.1. Effect of CO_2-enriched air on the yield and nitrogen content of field-grown soybeans.[a]

	Air (0.03 percent CO_2)	Enriched air (0.06 percent CO_2)
Dry weight (in grams per plant)		
Plant body	11.8	15.0
Seed pods	8.8	15.7
Nitrogen content (in grams per plant)		
Plant body	0.27	0.30
Seed pods	0.38	0.70
Nitrogen in the plants (in kilograms per hectare)		
Total	295	511
Obtained from the soil	219	84
Obtained from the nitrogen-fixing bacteria	76	427

[a]From R. W. F. Hardy and U. D. Havelka, paper presented at meeting on "Nitrogen Fixation and the Biosphere" held at Edinburgh, Scotland, 1973. Reprinted with permission.

of photosynthate (sugar) to these microorganisms greatly increases their ability to fix nitrogen for the soybean plants.

Temperature is another important environmental variable which affects the rate not only of photosynthesis but of all cellular processes; as a result, it has a profound influence on the rate of plant growth. Photosynthesis and growth proceed very slowly at low temperatures (below 7°C), and speed up as the temperature rises. Cellular processes such as photosynthesis usually proceed most efficiently at a certain optimal temperature. The optimal temperature for photosynthesis for most crop plants is between 20°C and 35°C, but there are large differences between species in this characteristic. Photosynthesis is slowed down when the air temperature exceeds the optimum temperature, and high temperatures (45° to 50°) are invariably detrimental to the growth of most crop plants. Respiration, which burns up the products of photosynthesis, proceeds optimally at 35° to 45°. There is therefore less net plant growth when the temperature exceeds the range which is optimal for photosynthesis, as is shown by Figure 4.5: notice that respiration continues to increase, but photosynthesis does not, when the temperature is increased above 25°. As a result, net plant growth is reduced above 25°. These facts show why most crop plants grow better if high daytime temperatures alternate with low nighttime temperatures. At night there is no

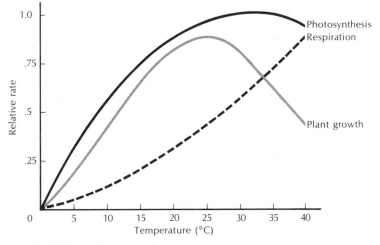

FIGURE 4.5.
Effect of temperature on photosynthesis, respiration, and the net accumulation of dry matter by the plant.

photosynthesis, but respiration continues; much of the sugar made during the day can be lost at night if the temperature remains high. Certain crops, such as potatoes and sugar beets, which must synthesize large amounts of carbohydrate in a short time, cannot be grown in areas where the night temperatures are high in the summer. The balance between photosynthesis and respiration appears to be one of the factors limiting plant growth in the tropics, where the temperatures do not drop during the night in the same way that they do in the temperate zones.

The distribution of water within the plant also affects the photosynthetic process. Although the photosynthetic fixation of CO_2 requires water, the amount of water used is very small in comparison to the total amount of water present in the plant. If there is not enough water in the leaves, the stomates will close and the leaves will wilt. Closure of the stomates prevents the diffusion of CO_2 into the leaf; so photosynthesis can not take place. The slight dehydration of the leaf cells which accompanies wilting also decreases the activities of the enzymes involved in the biochemical reactions of photosynthesis. Many crop plants undergo a period of temporary wilting in the early afternoon of hot days, even though there is an abundance of soil water, because water cannot be absorbed by the roots fast enough to keep up with water loss by evaporation from the leaves. This is the cause of the characteristic midday "slump" in the photosynthetic rate of many crop plants.

Minerals are important in many of the biochemical reactions of photosynthesis. The lack of certain minerals causes the plants to be pale green, indicating that they do not have sufficient chlorophyll. For example, magnesium is part of the chlorophyll molecules; iron is part of one of the primary acceptors of the energy absorbed by chlorophyll; and manganese plays an important role in the release of oxygen. A short supply of any of these minerals leads to a severe lowering of the photosynthetic rate.

PLANT PRODUCTIVITY AND ENERGY TRANSFER

The plant uses the products of photosynthesis to manufacture a variety of complex organic molecules, some of which have great nutritional value for human beings, and some of which have none. If glucose is made into cellulose—and most of the dry matter of a plant is cellulose and other cell-wall components—it does not benefit human beings directly. But if the glucose is made into starch, it may constitute an important food source. One way to increase food production is to increase the proportion of photosynthate that is channeled into starch, by breeding plants which produce more and larger seeds. Another way is to maximize plant productivity, the amount of CO_2 a plant fixes into photosynthetic products, because increased productivity usually leads to increased crop yield in the form of either starch or protein.

The Efficiency of Photosynthesis

One way to increase plant productivity is to maximize photosynthesis. This is a major aim of agricultural practice and of modern plant breeding. Photosynthesis is basically an energy-conversion process, and such processes are usually not very efficient. In an automobile, only about 20 percent of the chemical energy in gasoline is actually used as mechanical energy in running the engine. The rest is dissipated as heat or lost in an unusable form. Photosynthesis, being a conversion of light energy to chemical energy, is also not 100 percent efficient. About 2,500 Calories of sunlight are required by the plant to link together six molecules of CO_2 into a molecule of sugar, which contains about 700 Calories. Thus photosynthesis converts about 28 percent of the trapped light energy into chemical energy. However, the leaf usually cannot use all the sunlight impinging on it. On a summer day, only 20 percent of the available light can be used by a leaf even at peak photosynthetic efficiency. Thus, this peak efficiency, expressed in terms of the percentage of incoming light energy that is converted into energy contained in glucose, is 20 percent times 28 percent or approximately 5.6 percent. This is the *maximum* proportion of radiant energy that a photosynthetic system—a field of corn or a forest—can convert into chemical energy. This maximum could only be achieved, in theory, if very efficient plants were grown under ideal conditions. In practice, the efficiency of crop plants is closer to 1 to 3 percent.

Gross and Net Productivity

A second way to maximize plant productivity is to minimize the amount of energy that, after being fixed during photosynthesis, is used up by the plant itself and so not available for human use. The amount of energy which actually ends up in plant products (starch, cellulose, protein, etc.) is called the *net productivity* of the plant. It is usually much less than the *gross productivity*, which is the total amount of energy fixed during photosynthesis.

These two terms, gross and net productivity, can be applied not only to single plants, but also to entire ecosystems. The annual net productivity of an ecosystem is the amount of dry matter produced by plants each year. The two processes that reduce gross productivity are respiration and photorespiration.

Respiration takes place continually in both plants and animals. Its over-all effect is to reverse the equation for photosynthesis, so that the CO_2 that has been fixed is returned to the air. The amount by which respiration reduces the gross productivity of a plant varies considerably, from 20 percent in wheat to 40 percent in rice. In the African rain forest, 75 percent of the gross productivity is lost by respiration. But because respiration is essential for providing the plant with the energy necessary for its activities, there is not much human beings can do to lower this term in the equation.

During the day, plants such as wheat, rice, and soybeans respire away much of their fixed CO_2 by a process that is biochemically distinct from respiration. This process is activated by light, and is therefore called photorespiration. Up to half the products of photosynthesis are broken down directly into CO_2 by this process (see Figure 4.6). The role of photorespiration in plant growth is not known: however, since some plants with high net productivities (such as corn and sugarcane) exhibit little photorespiration, it is believed that photorespiration, unlike normal respiration, does not give energy to the plant in a form that it can use to drive its energy-requiring processes. When photorespiration is chemically blocked, net productivity

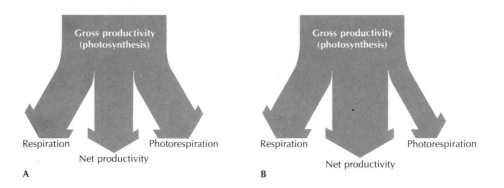

FIGURE 4.6.
A comparison of the use of photosynthetic products in two different species of plants. Species A, with high photorespiration, has less net productivity than species B, which has low photorespiration.

Table 4.2. Productivity of a tobacco leaf in light.[a]

	Grams of CO_2 fixed per square centimeter per hour
Gross productivity	4.7
Respiration loss	0.6
Photorespiration loss	2.6
Net productivity	1.5
Net productivity when photo-respiration is blocked chemically	4.1

[a]From I. Zelitch, *Photosynthesis, Photorespiration, and Plant Productivity* (Academic Press, 1971), p. 180.

rises dramatically. Table 4.2 shows data taken from an experiment with tobacco plants. The development of crop plants that do not undergo photorespiration would lead to an increased net productivity.

The net productivities of plants in nature differ greatly, largely because of environment. The arctic tundra and the desert have very low net productivities (100 to 200 grams of dry matter per square meter per year) whereas tropical forests have net productivities of 5,000 grams per square meter per year or even more. Productivity appears to be limited primarily by the amount of water that is available and by the amount of solar energy received. Calculations of the efficiency of energy conversion show that natural ecosystems convert from 0.1 to 1.8 percent of the sun's energy into chemical energy stored in plant products. In many areas plants do not grow year round, because it is either too dry or too cold; so the amount of light received during the growing season is often much less than the total amount of light received during the year. When efficiency of energy conversion is calculated in terms of light received during the growing season, it is found that natural ecosystems can convert from 0.2 to 3.5 percent of the incident solar energy into net productivity. However, well-managed agricultural systems, especially those consisting of tropical grasses and their cultivated relatives, such as corn and sugarcane, can be even more productive than natural ecosystems. They can convert up to 4.2 percent of the sunlight received during the growing period into dry matter.

Energy Transfer

The living world comprises many kinds of organisms, which do not live independently of one another, but instead interact with each other. How energy and matter are transferred between organisms is an important

Table 4.3. Food chains.

Trophic level	Land	Ocean	Farm
Producers	grasses	algae	grasses
Primary consumers	rabbit	zooplankton	cow
Secondary consumers	coyote	anchovy	humans
		herring	
		tuna	

aspect of the science of ecology. The organisms that are related by consumption of energy and matter are said to form a *food chain*.

In a food chain, organisms that share the same general source of nutrition are at the same trophic level. Green plants, which get their energy from the sun and their nutrition from the air and soil, form the first trophic level: the *producers*. The molecules (such as starch and proteins) that are made by plants become nutrition for organisms that feed on the producers: these are *consumers*. The first trophic level of consumers comprises the herbivores, organisms that feed exclusively on plants. The next levels contain carnivores, predatory animals which eat other animals (see Table 4.3). In addition to producers and consumers, a food chain also has *decomposers*. These organisms, of which many bacteria and fungi are examples, obtain their energy from dead organic matter. In a system where the producers and consumers are rapidly depleting the environment of nutrients, such as minerals, decomposers play a key role, by returning these nutrients to the environment in a form that the producers can use.

Animals, whether herbivores or carnivores, use food energy for a variety of purposes. Most of it is released in respiration to sustain energy-requiring activities of muscles and nerves and of many metabolic reactions. Only a small portion of the chemical energy which is taken in is retained within the body and is available as food for the next level of consumers (see Figure 4.7). On the average, about 90 percent of the energy taken in is respired away, and only 10 percent is stored. We have already mentioned that meat is an ecological luxury because the transfer of protein from producer (the corn plant) to consumer (the cow) is inefficient in terms of the amount of protein available for human consumption. Several (4 to 6) kilograms of cereal or other protein are needed to produce one kilogram of beef protein, because much of the protein that the cow eats is used for its biological functions. Only a small amount is used for making the structural proteins that human beings eat.

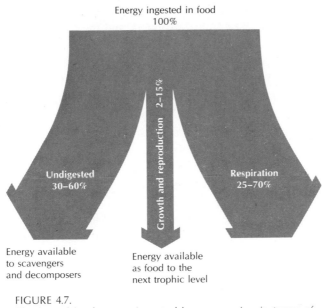

FIGURE 4.7.
The fate of food energy ingested by an organism in terms of the energy available for organisms at the next trophic level.

Agricultural scientists have attempted to increase the efficiency of these food chains by restricting the energy expenditure of the primary consumers and by selecting consumers which use much of their energy to make food. Efficiencies of energy transfer on feed lots now range up to 30 percent for feed grain to chickens. Another major difference between an agricultural and a natural system is that, in the agricultural system, one part of the food chain (producers) is favored over all others. Human beings modify the environment by irrigation, fertilization, and weed control to increase the net productivity of certain plants as much as possible, then keep away competing herbivores and divert the net productivity for their own use. Less energy is available to the decomposers because large amounts of organic matter are removed from the fields.

An Energy Budget for the World

Given the preceding considerations of productivity and energy transfer, we can calculate how many people the Earth can support at our present level of agricultural technology. To make such calculations, we must make certain assumptions about the amount of arable land available for food production, the productivity of the land, the desire of many people to consume large amounts of animal products, and the lifestyle of the people.

How many hectares are needed to support one person? A person who requires 2,700 Calories per day (an average figure) needs about 1,000,000 Calories per year. The productivity of many well-managed wheat-producing areas is around 4,000 kilograms per hectare. This corresponds to a net primary productivity of about 1,500 grams of dry matter per square meter per year. The grain yield is less than the primary productivity, because only 25 to 33 percent of the whole plant is grain. One kilogram of grain has a caloric content of 3,500 Calories and the wheat harvest mentioned above thus yields about 14 million Calories per hectare. As a result, one hectare can support fourteen people on a strictly vegetarian diet.

Many people want to eat large amounts of animal products. In many technologically advanced countries, animal products are produced largely by using grains which could be eaten by human beings. The efficiency of converting plant products to animal products is about 20 percent. Thus, if a person derives half his energy and protein from animal products, he will need a much larger area to support himself. Half the 1,000,000 Calories annually required will come from animals, and these 500,000 will use up 2,500,000 Calories in plant products. Such a person requires a total of three million Calories of plant products each year. Under these conditions, a hectare of land will support only four to five people.

Estimates of the arable land in the world range from three to four billion hectares. One of the most careful estimates, carried out by the Dutch crop physiologist C. T. deWit, arrives at a figure of only 2.3 billion hectares. All this land is now available for crop production, but some of it will become unavailable if the Earth's population continues to rise. This decline may occur for two reasons. Increasing population pressures on the Earth's resources often result in poor management of the existing agricultural land. Many areas are being overgrazed and overcropped, and too little is being done to maintain the fertility and structure of the soil. Destruction of vegetation may cause the topsoil to be blown away. An expansion of the population also diminishes the available crop land, because cities, highways, airfields, reservoirs, and ports are often built on agricultural land. How much agricultural land is lost in this way as the population expands depends very much on the lifestyle of the people. Estimates vary from one hectare for every three people added (in the sprawling cities of the U.S.) to one hectare for every 40 people (in densely crowded cities).

Using an average figure of one hectare of farmland in nonfarm use for every 12 people, we calculate that the world can support about 15 billion people on a vegetarian diet or 5 billion people on a mixed diet. Since the world population passed 4 billion in 1976, and will probably double within less than 35 years, the need for population control is apparent. Since these estimates of food production assume that maximal use is being made of the arable land, the need for widespread use of modern agricultural techniques and of high-yielding crop strains is also apparent.

CHAPTER 5 Nutrition from the Soil

Plants are the primary producers in all food chains, including those which lead to human beings. Plant productivity results from photosynthesis. In order to perform photosynthesis and other metabolic processes, land plants must extract water and minerals from the soil. Thus the soil is a "placenta of life," for it supplies nutrients to the plants, which in turn supply nutrients to all the organisms whose lives depend on plants. Throughout history, man's standard of living has depended on the water content, fertility, and productivity of the soil. Many people are hungry today because land that once was fertile can no longer support crop production, largely because of man's poor understanding of the nature of soils.

WATER

Water is the medium in which soil minerals are dissolved, and therefore it must be present in order for these nutrients to enter the roots of plants. This important role of soil water, however, cannot explain the extremely high water requirements of many crops. For an explanation of these requirements, we must consider the role of CO_2 in the leaf during photosynthesis.

Photosynthesis requires a continuous diffusion of CO_2 from the atmosphere into the leaf. This diffusion occurs through the stomates, tiny pores which dot the surface of the leaf. Photosynthesis can occur only if these pores are open and CO_2 can enter the leaf.

These open stomates also allow water vapor to escape from the interior air spaces of the leaf into the atmosphere. The water vapor in the intercellular spaces is quickly replenished by the evaporation of water from the leaf cells. The water evaporates because the leaf absorbs much more solar energy than it can use in photosynthesis. This energy must be dissipated, or it would heat the leaf to a temperature (50°C or more) which would kill the cells. The plant dissipates this heat partially by allowing the water in the leaf cells to become water vapor in the intercellular spaces. However, the leaf cells must replenish their water supply. Therefore they obtain water from the conductive tissues, which in turn get their water from the soil via the roots. Thus during the daytime, when the stomates are open, there is a continuous stream of water through the plant. This process is called *transpiration* (see Figure 5.1). At night, when the stomates are closed, the transpiration stream stops, although the plant may continue to take up water until it has become completely rehydrated.

Transpiration dissipates heat in plants much as perspiration does in humans. It also helps to transport minerals taken up from the soil, and organic substances made in the roots, throughout the plant. If the rate of water uptake from the soil is inadequate to replenish the water lost from the leaves by transpiration, the leaves will wilt, and this will cause the stomates to close. Closure of stomates prevents further water loss, but it also

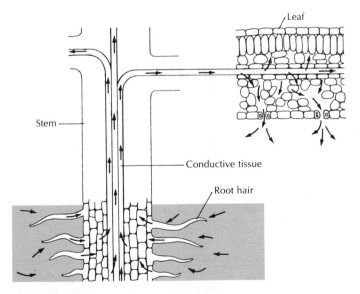

FIGURE 5.1.
The transpiration stream through a plant. Arrows indicate the direction of movement of water or water vapor.

prevents photosynthesis, since CO_2 cannot enter the leaf. On a hot summer day, plants may experience transient wilting, because water loss is more rapid than water uptake, even though there is sufficient water in the soil. This transient wilting can severely depress photosynthesis in midday. Thus provision of adequate soil water is crucial to plant productivity.

Many crop plants use large amounts of water. It has been calculated that a single corn plant in its growing season transpires about 200 liters of water. This means that a hectare of corn uses an amount of water equivalent to a layer measuring one hectare in surface and 25 cm in thickness. However, water is lost not only by transpiration, but also by evaporation from the soil surface. The sun warms the soil and causes some of the water to escape as water vapor. The term *evapotranspiration* describes the total amount of water which is lost from a plant-soil system. The total productivity of a system is very closely tied to the amount of water which is lost each year by evapotranspiration (see Figure 5.2). The availability of water in the soil determines plant growth more than any other factor.

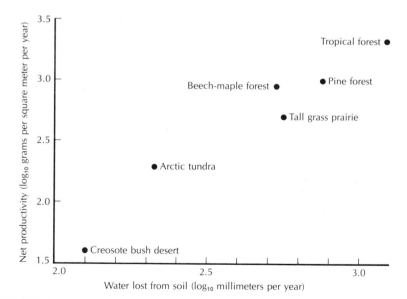

FIGURE 5.2.
The relationship between the water lost from the soil (by evaporation and transpiration) and plant productivity. In general, it is possible to predict productivity from data on temperature and water availability. (Adapted from M. Rosenzweig, "Net Primary Productivity of Terrestrial Communities: Prediction from Climatological Data," American Naturalist, 102, 1968, 67–74.)

Table 5.1. Water-use efficiencies.

Plant	Kilograms of water used per kilogram of dry matter produced
Alfalfa	850
Soybeans	650
Oats, potatoes	580
Wheat	550
Sugar beets	380
Corn	350
Sorghum	300

Plants differ in their water requirements. Different crops require different amounts of water, and this amount often determines where these plants can be grown. Some examples of the transpiration ratio, the number of kilograms of dry matter produced per kilogram of water evaporated, are given in Table 5.1. These are only approximate figures, because the water requirements of any plant depend on its environment and nutrition. When plants are grown in nutrient-rich soil, they are usually large and have extensive root systems. The total amount of water lost by transpiration increases, but the transpiration ratio declines. In one experiment with corn plants, the transpiration ratio of corn grown on poor soil was 2,000, but it declined to 350 when the soil was well fertilized. Thus, the larger, healthier plants used more water, but they used it more efficiently, producing more dry matter and more corn per kilogram of water extracted from the soil. Placing plants closer together increases the total transpiration, because there are more plants, but it decreases direct evaporation of water from the soil, because the sun does not hit the soil directly. In an experiment, the number of corn plants per hectare was increased from 20,000 to 40,000. This increased the corn yield by 65 percent, but the total loss of water from the soil by only 20 percent.

The water which is lost from the soil to the atmosphere by evapotranspiration must be replenished by precipitation and percolation of the water into the deeper layers of the soil. Agricultural production can only continue if the annual precipitation and percolation equals the annual evapotranspiration. Water loss from the soil during the growing season often exceeds water recharge, but the reverse is true in winter. Figure 5.3 shows the annual water loss by evapotranspiration, and water gain from precipitation, in the subsoil of the cornfield. Many of the soil-tilling activities of the

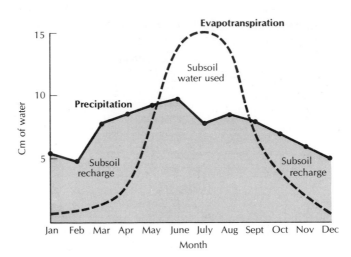

FIGURE 5.3.
Rainfall (lines connecting dots) and monthly water loss by crop growth and evaporation in the midwestern U.S.A. Note that rainfall during the growing season is not adequate for the needs of the plants, and they must use water stored in the soil. (From S. Aldrich and E. Leng, Modern Corn Production, *F and W Publishing, 1969, p. 171.)*

farmer are aimed at ensuring that the water which falls on the land will percolate into the subsoil rather than be lost as runoff. In dry areas, such tilling may mean the difference between success and failure in crop production.

SOILS

Soil Formation

The formation of a soil is a long and complex process, involving the breakdown of the parent rock into small mineral particles, the chemical modification of these particles, and finally the continuous addition and decomposition of organic residues from plants, animals, and microorganisms. Solid rock is continually being broken down into small particles, a process termed weathering. Weathering results from both physical and chemical forces. Even the hardest rocks can be fractured, in time, by alternate heating and cooling of the rock itself or by the freezing and thawing of water which seeps into cracks. Other physical forces which contribute to soil formation are running water, the scouring action of winds carrying small particles, and glaciers, which creep over the rocks, grinding them into small particles.

During the ice ages, this last process began forming what are now rich agricultural soils in many areas of the world.

Physical forces break up rocks into smaller particles, but chemical forces can change the chemical properties of these particles. The more a rock is fractured by physical weathering, the faster chemical weathering will occur. The Earth's crust contains more than 90 different elements, which can form certain combinations called minerals. These minerals usually form small crystalline grains, which are cemented together to form rocks. Many minerals are combinations of silicon, aluminum, iron, and oxygen, because these four elements are by far the most abundant in the Earth's crust. A simple granite, for example, may contain three different minerals: feldspar, mica, and quartz (see Table 5.2), which can be recognized as three different types of crystalline grains within it. During physical weathering the granite breaks up into its component mineral grains. This process is aided by rainwater, because the different mineral grains and the cementing substances are soluble in water to different degrees. Rainwater is not pure water, because it contains dissolved carbon dioxide, which forms carbonic acid. Although carbonic acid is a weak acid, it attacks the rocks more vigorously than water does.

Once the original minerals have been released, their proportions in the soil are greatly affected by temperature, rainfall, and vegetation. Some of them, such as quartz, are not changed, but are simply broken into smaller and smaller particles, whereas others such as feldspar or mica, are modified. Feldspar reacts with the carbonic acid and forms soluble potassium carbonate and kaolinite, or clay mineral. Mica is even further degraded. It falls apart into potassium carbonate, oxides of iron and aluminum, and clay. This complete dissolving of certain components of the mineral particles is an important aspect of the entire weathering process. Indeed, the minerals must be dissolved before they can be taken up by plants. Once the minerals

Table 5.2 Some primary minerals.

Mineral group	Typical composition
Mica	$KH_2Al_3(SiO_4)_3$
Feldspar	$KAlSi_3O_8$
Quartz	SiO_2
Iron oxide	Fe_2O_3
Carbonate	$CaCO_3$

have been dissolved, they can either remain in solution, or become bound to the outside surface of the soil particles, or react with other dissolved minerals to form insoluble compounds.

Soil formation depends not only on weathering but also on the simultaneous accumulation of the soil particles. Both water and wind can carry soil particles from their site of formation to other regions. For example, some of the soils that are the most agriculturally important today were formed 10,000 years ago, when winds deposited enormous amounts of clay and silt particles in certain areas. Others were formed at the end of the most recent ice age, when streams flowing from the melting glaciers deposited the particles; when the climate became drier, winds created great dust storms, depositing the particles over large areas of the world. But just as these factors form soils, so they can remove them, in the process of erosion. Plants play an important role in preventing erosion, because their roots hold the soil together, a lesson painfully learned in Oklahoma and Texas during the "dust bowls" of the 1930's.

Soil formation may occur rapidly or slowly, depending on the nature of the parent rock, the weather, the vegetation, and the topography. Flatlands with a warm, humid climate, a forest vegetation, and a parent rock which is easily broken down favor rapid soil formation. High rainfall and high temperatures promote rapid chemical weathering, because the dissolved mineral components are carried away to lower layers of the soil by the downward movement of water and because chemical reactions go faster at higher temperatures. The percolating water also leaches acids out of the decaying plant residues. The leachates from the decaying needles of conifers are more acid than those of the leaflitter in deciduous forests which in turn are more acid than the decay products of prairie grasses. Thus the type of vegetation affects chemical weathering.

Percolating rainwater causes dissolved minerals, bits of organic matter, and the smallest mineral particles to be slowly redistributed in the soil. This process, called leaching, is one of the most important in the formation of a mature soil. Once formed, a mature soil usually shows at least three distinct layers or *horizons* (see Figure 5.4). The A horizon, or topsoil, is the layer richest in the decaying organic matter and dissolved minerals that sustain plant growth. On the average, it is no more than 20 to 30 cm thick, but human survival on earth is intimately linked with the preservation of this very thin layer (on a 24-inch globe, the topsoil would be three millionths of an inch thick). Below the topsoil is the B horizon, or subsoil. Minerals

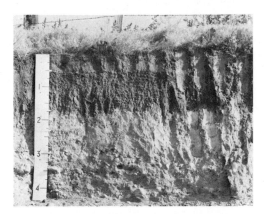

FIGURE 5.4.
A soil in profile, showing the different horizons. The scale is in feet. (Photo courtesy of U.S.D.A.)

leached out of the A horizon accumulate here. Most of a plant's roots are in the topsoil, but good farming practice often involves breaking up the subsoil to allow the plants to find additional water and nutrients. The third layer, or C horizon, consists of parent rock in the process of being broken up.

Soil Texture and Structure

The soil particles formed by the weathering of the parent material are not uniform in size, and can be classified according to their size as sand, silt, and clay. Sand particles range in diameter from 2 mm (millimeters) to 0.02 mm, and silt particles from 0.02 to 0.002 mm; all particles smaller than 0.002 mm are called clay particles. Soil scientists classify soils into different types according to the proportion of sand, silt, and clay particles each soil contains (see Table 5.3). These proportions, generally referred to

Table 5.3. Composition of three typical soils according to the size of the mineral particles.

Soil type	Type of particle		
	Sand	Silt	Clay
Sandy loam	85%	6%	9%
Loam	59	21	20
Clay	10	22	68

as the texture of a soil, are determined by the nature of the parent material and by the extent to which the minerals have been weathered. Sandy soils are often formed on sandstone, whereas limestone gives rise to loam soils; shale is more likely to result in clay-rich soils than either sandstone or limestone.

The sand and silt particles play an important role in the movement of air and water in the soil, whereas the clay particles enable the soil to bind and store water and nutrients. Both water and nutrients are *adsorbed* on the surface of the soil particles. Obviously, the more finely divided the particles, the greater their surface area per unit mass, and the greater their capacity to bind water and nutrients. Clay particles have often been weathered to such an extent that they become porous and so present an even greater binding surface. Thus sandy soils, having relatively more large particles, do not bind much water or plant nutrients in comparison to clay soils, which can bind enormous amounts of water and nutrients.

The individual soil particles are generally clumped together to form larger aggregates of varying size and shape. This is especially common with the smaller silt and clay particles. The "glue" that sticks the particles together is a combination of lime, hydroxides of iron, and humus and other decaying organic matter. The degree of aggregation of the particles is generally referred to as the structure or *tilth* of the soil. Although soil structure is difficult to define, it is readily recognized from the size and shape of the lumps which are formed when a soil is crumbled.

For agriculture the tilth of a soil is more important than its texture. The soil's suitability for plant growth depends on the tilth, because of the pore spaces which exist between the soil particles and the aggregates. These pores, which occupy about half a soil's volume, can contain air, or water, or both. Roots need both air and water, and the ratio of air to water in the pore space is affected by the tilth of the soil.

Air and Water

The size of the individual pores in the soil is related to the size of the particles or aggregates. Small pores normally occur between small particles, whereas larger pores exist between large particles or aggregates. The small pores, called capillaries, are usually filled with water, whereas the larger ones are filled with air. A good, fertile soil should have half the pore space filled with water and the other half with air. Such a distribution provides a good balance between aeration, water percolation, and water-storage capacity.

The importance of air for plant roots and for most other soil organisms is commonly underestimated. Plant roots need energy to grow and to take up minerals, and they obtain this energy by respiring the sugars made in the leaves. This respiration requires oxygen and causes CO_2 to be given off. To maintain the proper balance of oxygen and carbon dioxide in the soil, there must be continuous movement of the gases in and out of the soil. Oxygen from the atmosphere must move into the soil, and carbon dioxide must be allowed to escape, or it will build up to toxic levels. This movement of gases requires that continuous air channels be present in the soil. Such channels are made by small burrowing animals, such as worms, or are formed when dead plant roots decay. Gas exchange between the atmosphere and the soil readily occurs when the soil has an adequate proportion of large pores as well as a system of channels.

To understand how water behaves in the soil, consider what happens to dry soil during a prolonged slow rainfall or watering. As soon as the water touches the soil particles and organic matter, it binds to them. The water molecules nearest the particle are held with the greatest force and cannot be dislodged from the particle. The rest of the water fills the smaller pores and percolates downward through the larger pores. This binding process is then repeated for the lower soil particles. A soil which becomes saturated with water in this way is said to be at field capacity: all the small pores are filled with water, but the large pores are filled with air. If enough water falls on the soil and if percolation is adequate, it may eventually become saturated down to the underground water table. If still more water is added, these underground reservoirs will rise. Now water fills not only the small pores but also the large ones. When this filling of air spaces reaches to top layers of a soil, it becomes waterlogged. A waterlogged soil literally suffocates most plants and soil organisms. They die for lack of air.

The texture and structure of a soil together determine how well it can store water and whether the water will be able to percolate through the soil (see Table 5.4). A clay soil, with its preponderance of small particles, has many small pores and a large water-storage capacity. There may be so few large pores, however, that water cannot percolate downward. Rain-water then gathers on the surface of the soil and eventually runs off, often taking the vital topsoil with it. Adding organic matter to such soils causes

Table 5.4. Water-holding capacities of different soils.

Soil type	Cm of available water[a] per 30 cm of soil
Coarse sand	1.25
Very fine sand	3.00
Very fine sandy loam	4.75
Silt loam	5.25
Silty clay	6.50
Clay	7.00

[a]Water that plants can take up from the soil.

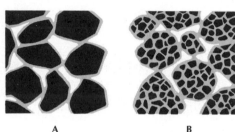

A   B

FIGURE 5.5.
Schematic representation of water and air in sandy (A) and clay (B) soils. In sand, there are larger air spaces but less water adhering to the soil particles. In clay, the particles aggregate, and most of the spaces between them are filled with water.

the formation of aggregates, which create larger pores, causing more rapid percolation. Maintaining plant cover on the land thus helps to prevent erosion in two different ways: the roots of the plants stabilize the topsoil, thereby preventing it from being carried away; and the decaying plants also supply the organic matter necessary for aggregate formation, causing more rapid percolation.

Soil Organisms

The soil is not a static system consisting of inert components, but rather a dynamic community in which energy and matter are continually being converted from one form into another. These conversions depend on the activities of the soil organisms. Most soils contain a great variety of organisms, from the microscopic viruses and bacteria to the large burrowing mammals (see Table 5.5), and each group plays its own role in the soil. Except for the green algae and certain autotrophic bacteria, all the soil organisms depend on the photosynthetic activities of the plants to pro-

Table 5.5. Soil organisms.[a]

Organism type	Amount in fertile soil (kilograms per hectare)
Bacteria	800
Fungi	3,300
Protozoa	330
Algae	275
Worms, insects	1,020

[a]Modified from T. Brock, *Principles of Microbial Ecology* (Prentice-Hall, 1966), p. 3.

vide them with a source of food energy. In Chapter 4 we saw that the decomposers are a group of organisms which play an important role in the flow of energy and nutrients in many food chains. Decomposers are microorganisms which use dead organic matter as their source of food. They are found primarily in the soil, where they cause nutrients to be released from the organic matter so that these nutrients can then be used again by growing plants.

The bacteria are by far the most numerous organisms in the soil, and they are of great importance in a variety of soil processes. A gram of fertile soil may contain more than a billion bacteria, equivalent to a live weight of more than 3,000 kg per hectare. Infertile soils contain fewer bacteria, but the fertility of a soil can, unfortunately, not be predicted by simply counting the number of bacteria per gram of soil. Most soil bacteria are small rod-shaped organisms measuring less than 1 micron in width and a few microns in length (one micron is 10^{-6} meter). Many swim around actively in the soil solution. When conditions are favorable, bacteria can multiply very rapidly. Some divide as often as once every hour, although others take much longer. Rapid rates of multiplication can be maintained only when there is adequate food. When the nutrients are exhausted, the populations decrease; many bacteria form spores, which can lie dormant in the soil until conditions for growth are favorable.

There are both autotrophic and heterotrophic bacteria in the soil. The heterotrophic bacteria can use a wide variety of organic molecules as their source of food. They degrade these molecules and ingest the products to build up their own structures. In the process, they absorb nutrients, such as ammonia, nitrate, sulfate, or phosphate, which are also needed by plants. Fortunately for man, these heterotrophic bacteria also degrade many of the organic herbicides and pesticides which are now used in large quantities. Some of these compounds are degraded very slowly, however, and may accumulate in the soil.

Several species of bacteria are able to use atmospheric nitrogen (N_2) in the process of nitrogen fixation. Some of these invade plant roots, where they help the plant obtain nitrogen. The importance of this process is discussed later in this chapter.

The autotrophic bacteria are not as numerous in the soil as the heterotrophic ones, but they are involved in some important chemical transformations. The conversion of ammonium (NH_4^+) to nitrate (NO_3^-), and the oxidation of sulfide (S^{--}) to sulfate (SO_4^{--}), are carried out by different species of autotrophic bacteria.

The fungi, another class of organisms, are also important in contributing to soil processes and plant nutrition. In acidic soils they are more important than the bacteria, because they tolerate acidic conditions much better than most bacteria. Many fungi play an important role in the decomposition of organic matter in the soil. They secrete substances which break down the large organic molecules in the soil, releasing nutrients for themselves and for plants. Wood consists primarily of two types of large molecules: cellulose and lignin. The cellulose can be broken down by either bacteria or fungi, but only fungi can decompose the lignin. For this reason, fungi are the principal organisms responsible for the breakdown of woody tissues.

Some fungi secrete substances which can attack the cell walls of living plants. The small roots of young seedlings are particularly susceptible to fungus attack, and seeds are often coated with a fungicide before planting to prevent the fungal invasion which causes rootrot. Other fungi that invade plant roots establish a mutually beneficial relationship with the plant. The association between a root and a fungus is called a *mycorrhiza*. The threads of the fungus penetrate into the cells of the outer tissues of the root, and the fungus proliferates both inside the root and on the surface of the root. The plant furnishes the fungus with food in the form of photosynthetic products, and the fungus helps the plant obtain nutrients from the soil. Such mycorrhizas are often found in trees. In fertile soils they seem to have little effect on tree growth, but in infertile soils the tree derives great benefit from the presence of the fungus.

Important groups of larger soil animals are the nematodes (eelworms), the earthworms, and the insects. The smallest and most numerous of these are the nematodes. A cubic meter of topsoil may contain up to ten million nematodes. Some of these live off the dead organic matter; others parasitize plants and animals. The plant parasites usually have a very sharp mouthpiece with which they puncture the outer cells of the roots. They then invade the roots and start to multiply, causing the root tissues to swell. This renders the root system much less effective in taking up water and minerals and also directly damages root crops.

The beneficial effects of earthworms for plant growth are well known to home gardeners. Earthworms play an important role in aerating the soil and in mixing it, and in the decomposition of leaf litter. Some species of earthworms continually burrow through the soil, ingesting it and partially digesting the organic matter. In the process, soil particles become "glued" together to form stable aggregates, and the organic matter is transformed into humus. Other species of earthworms live near the surface of the soil and pull whole leaves into their burrows either to use them as food or to cover the entrance. The burrows themselves provide channels through which water can percolate into the soil and gases (oxygen or carbon dioxide) can diffuse.

Organic Matter

Organic matter in soils is derived from the residues of the plants and animals which live in and on the soil. Leaf litter accumulates on the soil surface in many forests; as it decays, it is gradually mixed with the top layer of soil (earthworms are especially important in this process) and carried downward by percolating water. In this way it becomes distributed through-out the A horizon. Organic residues are also contributed by the roots of plants (see Table 5.6) and by the soil organisms. The organic matter in the soil often gives it a characteristic brown color. Sandy soils and many

Table 5.6. The organic residues in the roots of crops grown in central Ohio under better than average conditions.

Crop	Kilograms of residue per hectare
Soybeans	600
Wheat	830
Corn	1,270
Alfalfa	3,850
Kentucky bluegrass	5,000

tropical soils are usually light-colored, because they contain very little organic matter (1 to 2 percent), whereas heavy clays can vary from dark brown to black, because they contain much more organic matter (5 to 10 percent).

The proportion of organic matter in a soil depends on the rate at which it is being added to the soil and the rate at which it is being broken down by the soil organisms. The rate of decay is very much influenced by the prevailing temperature, by the availability of oxygen, and by the acidity of the soil. The first phase of the decay process is carried out partly by earthworms and other soil animals, which ingest large amounts of leaf litter and dead roots. These materials are used as a source of food, and the animals excrete a black organic residue called humus. This process of transforming the organic residues into humus is aided by the soil microorganisms. Decay is carried out by organisms which require oxygen for their respiration. As a result, it usually proceeds much more rapidly in well-aerated soils.

The temperature and degree of acidity of the soil affect the decay of organic matter, because they influence microbial activity. High temperatures, as in the tropics, speed up the growth of microorganisms, which in turn speeds up decay (see Table 5.7). Acidic soils are usually rich in organic matter, because neither earthworms nor most bacteria can thrive in such soils; so decomposition of organic matter is slow. Although humus is more resistant to decay than fresh organic residues, it too is eventually broken down by microorganisms. The plant nutrients which it contains are then released into the soil and become available to the plants. The slow decay of humus provides the plants with a steady flow of nutrients, and is of great importance to soil fertility.

Table 5.7. Annual leaf production and turnover time for the organic matter in several ecosystems at different temperatures.[a]

System	Annual leaf production (kilograms per hectare)	Residual litter accumulation (kilograms per hectare)	Time for decay of organic matter (years)
Rainforest (tropical)	14,000	9,000	1.7
Deciduous forest (temperate)	4,500	14,000	4.0
Conifer forest (northern)	2,700	40,000	14.0
Tundra (Arctic)	900	45,000	50.0

[a]Data from various sources quoted by C. Kucera, *The Challenge of Ecology* (Mosby, 1973), p. 64.

To understand how the process of decomposition works, let us examine what happens when fresh organic matter, such as straw or a rich farm manure, is added to the soil. Immediately, the soil microorganisms start working on this organic matter, and, because they have this enormous source of food, they start to multiply rapidly. However, in addition to an energy source (provided by the carbohydrates), these organisms need nutrients to grow, especially nitrogen. If the organic matter has more nitrogen than the micro-organisms need for their own growth, nitrogen will be released into the soil by the decay processes. However, if the organic matter is poor in nitro-gen, the microorganisms will use up the nitrate already present in the soil, thereby robbing the plants of their source of nitrogen (see Figure 5.6). Since farmyard manure contains nitrogen-rich organic matter (animal wastes) and many mineral nutrients, its decay provides the plants with a steady

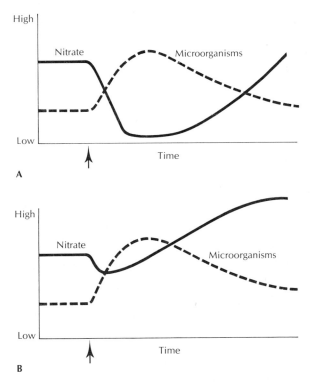

FIGURE 5.6.
Changes in the amount of soil nitrate (solid line) and the activity of decomposer microorganisms (dashed line) when nitrogen-poor (A) or nitrogen-rich (B) organic material is added to the soil (at the time indicated by the arrows). Note the more rapid release of increased nitrogen available to the plants in (B).

supply of nutrients. Straw and leaflitter are poor in nitrogen and minerals, and their decay may slow down plant growth, because plants and microorganisms are competing for the same nutrients. The setback for the plants is only temporary; eventually all these plant nutrients will be released back into the soil when the decomposition is complete and the population of microorganisms declines.

The conversion of a natural system to an agricultural one usually decreases the amount of organic matter in the soil, for several reasons. Tilling the soil and mixing the crop residues into the topsoil increases microbial activity because it increases the aeration of the topsoil. The addition of inorganic fertilizers provides the bacteria and fungi with the nutrients they need to decompose the crop residues more rapidly. Thus agriculture accelerates the decay of organic matter by causing an increase in microbial activity. This affects both the new crop residues and manures and the humus.

Some scientists have argued that this slow decline in the amount of organic matter in cultivated soils will eventually cause them to become useless for agriculture. The important factor in maintaining soil fertility is not the total amount of organic matter, but the amount of organic matter which is rapidly decaying. A large amount of rapidly decaying organic matter can be maintained in the soil by working crop residues into the soil regularly.

PLANT NUTRITION

The idea that plants need to take up minerals from the soil was experimentally documented for the first time in 1699 by the British botanist John Woodward. He grew small sprigs of mint in rainwater, river water, and water to which some soil had been added. When he weighed the mint plants some time later, he concluded that growth was related to the amount of dissolved substances in the water. To understand plant nutrition and the use of fertilizers to increase crop yields, we must look at the chemical elements which are actually *required* for plant growth, and at the ways in which the soil supplies the plants with these essential nutrients.

The Essential Elements

We saw earlier that the Earth's crust is made up of over ninety different chemical elements. An analysis of plant ash, the residue which remains after plants are burned, reveals that plants may take up as many as fifty or sixty different elements from the soil. Are all of these essential for growth, or does the plant take up whatever it happens to find in the soil? This question was first investigated in a systematic way in 1860 by the German plant physiologist Julius Sachs, who grew plants with their roots immersed in solutions of minerals. This technique is called water culture or hydroponics. He found that many plants could be grown satisfactorily in solutions containing only three mineral salts: calcium nitrate, potassium phosphate, and magnesium sulfate. These salts provided the plants with six elements: calcium, potassium, magnesium, nitrogen, sulfur and phosphorus, termed the major nutrient elements. If any one of these elements was omitted from the culture solution, the plants did not grow well, and Sachs concluded that these six elements were essential for the plant. These experiments also showed that plants did not require any organic substances (such as vitamins), a question which was hotly debated at the time.

Modern research suggests that the nutrient solutions used by Sachs were probably contaminated with small amounts of many other minerals. Advances in chemistry made it possible to obtain much purer chemicals, and it was shown during the first half of this century that plants also require trace amounts of six other minerals. These six, termed the minor nutrient elements, are boron, copper, chlorine, manganese, molybdenum, and zinc. Iron, already known to be essential by Sachs, is usually added to this list of minor nutrients.

These 13 major and minor nutrient elements are essential for the health of all plants. A few other elements are apparently needed by only some plants. Sodium is required by a number of plants which grow in salty environments. Diatoms, a major component of oceanic phytoplankton, and some cereals, such as rice, need silicon. The microorganisms which live in the roots of leguminous plants and fix nitrogen need cobalt. As a result, many legumes can only be successfully cultivated if the soil contains sufficient cobalt.

The other forty or fifty elements present in plant ash are taken up by the plants from the soil even though they may not be required for growth. This somewhat indiscriminate uptake of elements may benefit the animals which eat the plants. For example, animals require sodium and iodine, two elements not needed by plants. Plants may also accumulate elements which are toxic to animals. The "loco weed," which grows in the western U.S., accumulates the element selenium. This apparently does the plant no harm, but it kills the sheep, cattle, and horses which eat it.

Dissolved Minerals in the Soil Water

Chemical weathering causes mineral particles in the soil to slowly disintegrate. Some minerals dissolve easily, others more slowly, and still others precipitate out after they have been dissolved. The 13 essential elements or nutrients discussed above must be dissolved in the soil water before they can be taken up by the plants. Indeed, essential elements which are locked up in the mineral particles of the soil are unavailable to the plants until they enter the soil solution after the particles have been weathered. Thus the fertility of a soil depends on the extent to which the minerals have become dissolved and have remained in a usable form in the A and B horizons.

When minerals dissolve in water, they break up into smaller charged particles called ions. Ions with a positive electrical charge are termed cations; their negative counterparts are anions. Table 5.8 shows that the 13 essential elements occur in the soil as cations or anions. Whether an essential element is normally present in the soil as a cation or an anion is of agricultural importance, because the negatively charged ions are more easily leached out of the topsoil. To understand this, we must consider again the surface properties of the soil particles, both mineral and organic, which determine not only the soil's ability to bind water, but also its ability to bind many plant nutrients.

The mineral and organic soil particles have an over-all negative charge. Since opposite charges attract, cations bind to these particles. As a result, most of the cations in a soil are more or less firmly bound to the particles, although some remain in the soil solution. The anions, on the other hand, remain in the soil water. Because of their negative charge, they do not bind to the soil particles. As rainwater percolates through the soil, it carries anions and cations with it down to the groundwater. This process is called leaching. Since the anions are not bound to the soil particles, they are more easily

Table 5.8. Plant nutrients in soil water.

Element	Cation form in soil water	Element	Anion form in soil water
Calcium	Ca^{++}	Phosphorus	PO_4^{-3} (phosphate)
Magnesium	Mg^{++}	Sulfur	$SO_4^{=}$ (sulfate)
Potassium	K^+	Chlorine	Cl^- (chloride)
Manganese	Mn^{++}	Boron	BO_4^- (borate)
Iron	Fe^{++}	Molybdenum	$MoO_4^{=}$ (molybdate)
Copper	Cu^+	Nitrogen	NO_3^- (nitrate)
Zinc	Zn^{++}		
Nitrogen	NH_4^+ (ammonia)		

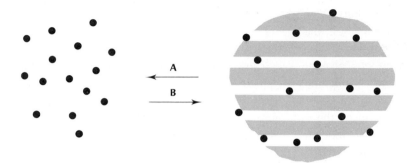

FIGURE 5.7.
Equilibrium between cations in the soil solution and those bound to the surface of clay particles. (A) Removal of nutrients by the roots from the soil solution causes more nutrients to leave the surface of the particles. (B) Addition of nutrients, in the form of fertilizer or from decay of organic matter, causes more nutrients to be bound to the clay particles.

lost by leaching than the cations, which are replenished as soon as they are removed. Indeed, as soon as cations are removed from the soil solution, either by leaching or because they are taken up by plants, they will be replaced by others which become unbound from the particles. Thus, there is an equilibrium between the cations in the soil water and those bound to the particles, as illustrated in Figure 5.7.

The total amount of available plant nutrients bound to soil particles is termed the soil's exchange capacity, a parameter which determines soil fertility. Because the surface area available for binding nutrients depends on texture, a soil's texture greatly influences its exchange capacity and its fertility. The greater the surface area of the particles, as in clay soils, the more plant nutrients they can bind. As water percolates down through the soil, it often carries nutrients down with it, especially the unbound anions, such as nitrate. In the groundwater, these nitrates may be quite abundant, and are dangerous if the groundwater is tapped for human drinking: as a result of heavy fertilization with nitrate, the groundwater in certain areas of Illinois and of the Central Valley of California is not fit for human consumption.

Acidity of the Soil Water

An important property of soil is its degree of acidity, which influences its physical properties, the availability of certain plant nutrients, and the biological activity in the soil. As a result, acidity strongly influences plant growth. The degree of acidity of a soil depends on the concentration of hydrogen ions (which have a positive charge) dissolved in the soil water. In a neutral soil, the hydrogen-ion concentration is about one part per ten million parts of water. Acidic soils contain a higher concentration of hydrogen ions, alkaline soils a lower concentration. Neither extreme acidity nor extreme alkalinity are suitable for the growth of plants and most other organisms. In addition, these conditions upset soil weathering and the availability of the nutrients. Although some plants can grow in heavily acidic or alkaline soils, most crop plants grow best in neutral or slightly acidic soils.

The minerals which are dissolved by chemical weathering can sometimes interact with each other to form new, insoluble complexes. The degree of acidity of a soil plays an important role in this process, which can greatly reduce the availability of certain nutrients to the plants. For example, phosphate, an essential plant nutrient, can form a variety of insoluble complexes with other ions in the soil solution. If the soil solution is too acidic, phosphate readily combines with calcium to form insoluble calcium phosphate. When the soil solution is slightly alkaline, phosphate combines with iron, aluminum, and manganese to form insoluble products. Thus phosphate is most readily available to plants when the soil solution is neutral or slightly acidic. The effect of the degree of acidity of the soil on some plant nutrients is shown in Figure 5.8.

The degree of acidity of a soil can be adjusted to make it more nearly neutral. Lime neutralizes excess acid in the soil, and acidic fertilizers, such as ammonium sulfate, neutralize excess alkalinity. Farmers may also use such treatments to optimize the growth of certain crops. For example, potatoes grow best in a somewhat acidic soil, whereas alfalfa thrives in a soil that is very slightly alkaline.

Uptake and Function of Minerals

In order to take up nutrients from the soil solution, most plants must develop an extensive root system. The root system provides the plant with the large surface area it needs to exploit a large volume of soil. In many plants this surface area is enormously increased by the presence of roothairs close to the tips of the roots. The ions absorbed from the soil by the root are in contact with the root surface, because they have moved through the soil or because the root has grown into a previously unexploited area. Which of these two processes is more important depends on the soil type and on the plant species. The rapid uptake of nutrients required by most crop plants

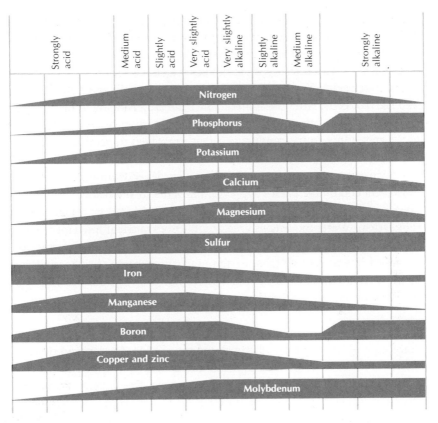

FIGURE 5.8.
The availability of nutrients to plants is affected by the condition of the soil. The more soluble a nutrient is, the thicker is the horizontal band representing the nutrient. Solubility in turn is directly related to the availability of the nutrient in an ionic form that is assimilable by the plant. Note that the best over-all balance is a slightly acidic soil. (From C. J. Pratt, "Chemical Fertilizers." Copyright © 1965 by Scientific American, Inc. All rights reserved.)

for maximal yield necessitates continuous growth by the root system. Much evidence indicates that the uptake from any one region of the soil has nearly ceased five or six days after it was first penetrated by a root.

Minerals do not pass into the outer root cells by passive diffusion, because the concentration of minerals is usually higher within the roots than in the soil water. Rather, they are "pulled" into the roothair cells by a process termed *active transport*. The word "active" is used because the ions are moving into the root against their natural tendency to diffuse out. This transport process requires energy, which comes from respiration in the root of sugars produced by photosynthesis in the leaves. The exact mechanism of active transport is not known, but special proteins located in the outer cell membrane may bind to the minerals and "escort" them into the root cells. After the mineral nutrients are inside the root cells, they pass from cell to cell until they reach the conductive tissues in the center of the root. Once in the conductive tissue, dissolved minerals can be transported throughout the plant.

Movement of nutrients within the plant depends on the rate of water movement and on the plant's supply of nutrients. If the plant is poorly supplied with nutrients, more of the entering nutrients will be retained in the root system. Water movement greatly influences nutrient movement within the plant, and the organs with the greatest rate of transpiration, the fully expanded leaves, receive most of the nutrients because they receive most of the water. Nutrients are needed most, however, by the growing parts of the plant, and consequently must be redirected from the mature leaves to the growing ones.

In many crop plants, seed maturation occurs at the same time as the senescence of the vegetative body of the plant: reproduction and death are linked in time. Root growth and nutrient uptake slow down at the onset of seed maturation. In bean plants, for example, the uptake of phosphate from the soil is not continuous throughout the cycle, but levels off once seed maturation begins. The accumulation of phosphate in the developing seeds occurs at the expense of the phosphate already present in the leaves and stem. Senescence and death of these vegetative organs is accompanied by a decline in their phosphate content. There are similar redistribution patterns for many other nutrients. This redistribution also involves a breakdown of the large organic molecules (e.g., proteins) and the transport of small organic molecules (e.g., amino acids) to the maturing seeds.

The various nutrients have specific roles in plants, which are often similar to their roles in animals. For example, plants require nitrogen and sulfur to synthesize amino acids, and they need phosphorus to make phospholipids and nucleic acids. Many minor nutrients, needed only in trace amounts, serve as cofactors for enzymes, much as they do in animals. Nutrients that have unique roles in plants include calcium, which participates in maintaining the integrity and rigidity of the cell wall, and magnesium, which is part of the chlorophyll molecule.

Nutrients also play an important role in maintaining the turgidity of the plant's organs. Plants actively take up ions from the soil, with the result that the total concentration of ions inside the root is greater than that outside. As a result of this difference in concentration, water moves from the soil solution into the roots, and thence to the rest of the plant. The difference in mineral concentration "drives" the uptake of water by the roots. The influx of water causes the cells to swell, and creates pressure within each cell. The water pressure acts as an internal skeleton, giving rigidity to cells and plant organs which lack strong cell walls. When water loss by evaporation exceeds water uptake, the pressure inside the cells drops. As a result, plant organs which lack strong cell walls (leaves, in many plants) do not retain their shape but collapse, and the plant wilts. Water pressure also drives cell enlargement in the growing zones of the plant, thus playing a key role in plant growth.

Deficiency Diseases and Fertilizers

If the soil is deficient in even one plant nutrient, plant growth will be retarded and the crop yield may be diminished. If the deficiency is severe, the plants will develop the visible symptoms of a deficiency disease. Such diseases are in many ways similar to those caused by the lack of vitamins or minerals in humans. Each disease is diagnostic of the element that is deficient. Modern farmers are familiar with the symptoms of the common deficiency diseases, and can recognize them when the plants are still young. Treatment usually involves fertilizing the soil with the deficient nutrient. Unless this is done at an early stage in plant growth, severe crop damage may occur.

The appearance of symptoms such as stunted growth, yellowing of the leaves, "burned" leaf margins, or death of the terminal bud usually indicates a rather severe deficiency in one or more plant nutrients. Plants do not develop these signs of deficiency when the nutrients are only marginally deficient: however, such marginal deficiencies may cause a large loss of crop yield. This "hidden hunger" is difficult to diagnose. It can sometimes be uncovered by measuring the amounts of plant nutrients in the soil or in the plant sap. Neither method is completely satisfactory, but reliable tests for measuring some of the important plant nutrients have been developed.

Although the total amounts of particular nutrients present in the soil can be measured, it is not possible to discover by chemical tests what proportion of the nutrients is available to the plants. Farmers, when deciding on a fertilizer program, are primarily interested in available nutrients. Availability can only be measured by experiments with plants. In spite of this problem, much progress has been made in developing soil tests which indicate the fertility of the soil. Agricultural scientists use the results of such tests to make recommendations to farmers about the use of fertilizers. The development of soil tests for available nutrients involves first of all, measuring how the yield of crop plants responds to the addition of fertilizers on a specific soil. After the yield responses are known, the plants are analyzed to measure how much of the nutrients they took up from the soil. This allows the soil chemists to develop analytical methods which accurately measure the available nutrients.

Nutrients in plant sap are on their way from the roots to leaves and seeds, where they will be used. Direct measurement of these nutrients in plants in the field can help diagnose potential crop troubles. It is not sufficient to make a single measurement. Rather, samples are taken every two weeks to find out how much of the nutrient is in the sap throughout the season. This method allows a farmer to diagnose hidden hunger before it actually affects crop production.

Soils can be deficient in plant nutrients for a variety of reasons. Harvesting crops removes large amounts of the major nutrients (see Table 5.9). These must be restored if the fertility of the soil is to be maintained. Failure to restore the nutrients leads to a gradual decline in soil fertility and crop productivity. This is adequately demonstrated by the low yields obtained

Table 5.9. Nutrients contained in the total above-ground plant material in a hectare of corn yielding 10,000 kg of grain.[a]

Nutrient	Kg/hectare	Nutrient	Kg/hectare
Nitrogen	200	Chlorine	86
Phosphorus	42	Iron	2.3
Potassium	205	Manganese	0.4
Calcium	41	Copper	0.1
Magnesium	48	Zinc	0.42
Sulfur	24	Boron	0.19
		Molybdenum	0.01

[a]From S. Barber and R. Olson, *Changing Patterns of Fertilizer Use* (Soil Science Society of America, 1968), by permission of the American Society of Agronomy.

on experimental plots which have not been fertilized for many years. Soils may appear to be deficient in certain nutrients because the nutrients are unavailable to the plants, as can happen when the soil is either too acid or too alkaline (shown in Figure 5.8). Highly weathered soils in tropical or semitropical areas can often be deficient in certain nutrients because leaching has removed them from the plant-root zone. The fact that such soils support a luxuriant vegetation does not necessarily indicate that they contain large amounts of available plant nutrients. Sandy soils are often deficient in certain nutrients, because they contain too small a proportion of clay particles, and are low in organic matter. As a result, they have a small exchange capacity, and thus a low fertility. Finally, soils may be deficient in nutrients because the parent material from which they developed contained only small amounts of certain nutrients, as sometimes happens for certain trace elements.

There are many ways to increase or restore the fertility of the soil so that it will support maximal crop production. One of the oldest methods is to allow the land to lie fallow for a long time. If no crops are grown and no plant nutrients are removed, the natural processes of soil weathering will slowly restore the fertility of the soil. The system of shifting agriculture practiced in the tropics is based on this principle. A second widely practiced method is to incorporate organic residues and wastes into the soil. A survey of agricultural practices around the world reveals that all kinds of organic residues are incorporated into the soil: manure, fish wastes, algae, human excrement, crop residues, sawdust, composted kitchen scraps, and many others. These organic fertilizers are decomposed in the soil and their nutrients are released. Organic fertilizers have the advantage that the plants can obtain a steady supply of nutrients, but have also the disadvantage that they may not release sufficient nutrients during the period of rapid vegetative growth, when demand is greatest. Slower growth in the early summer often means a reduced crop in the fall. It is a popular misconception that farmers in technologically advanced countries underestimate the value of organic fertilizers. The efforts made by most farmers to reincorporate the crop residues (leaves and stems in all seed crops) into the soil proves the opposite. Still, more could be done to compost the organic portion of household garbage, so that the plant nutrients contained in it could be used again by other plants.

A third method to restore the fertility of the soil is to add inorganic fertilizers (also called "chemical" or "synthetic" fertilizers). They offer the advantage that the nutrients are rapidly released and can be made available when the plant has the greatest need for them. A disadvantage is that some plant nutrients, especially nitrate, may be leached out of the root zone before the plants can use them. This problem is greatest if the fertilizers are applied just before or at the time of planting. It will take the seedlings several weeks to develop a root system large enough to take full advantage of the fertilizer.

The use of inorganic fertilizers to promote crop production is governed by two principles: the *law of the minimum* and the *law of diminishing returns*. The law of the minimum was first formulated in the nineteenth century by von Liebig, a German chemist who realized that plant growth is limited by the one nutrient which is in shortest supply in the soil. The addition of this nutrient will increase plant growth until some other nutrient becomes the limiting factor. However, plants differ in their nutrient requirements. Thus, the addition of phosphate to the soil is only beneficial to those plants for which phosphate is the limiting nutrient in the soil. If some other factor, such as water, light, or heat, limits the growth of the plant, then fertilizers will have no effect at all.

The second principle which governs the use of fertilizers was first formulated by E. A. Mitscherlich, another German scientist, who was concerned with the response of crop plants to added fertilizers. This principle, the law of diminishing returns, says that the amount of increase in the yield that is obtained from adding a given amount of fertilizer decreases as more and more fertilizer is added (see Figure 5.9). Adding 67 kg of nitrogen fertilizer per hectare caused wheat yields to increase by 4,700 kg per hectare. When another 67 kg of nitrogen per hectare was added, wheat yields increased still further, but the amount of increase was smaller (about 2,000 kg/ha). The addition of yet another 67 kg of nitrogen per hectare (for a total of 201 kg/ha) caused an even smaller increment of yield (700 kg/ha). These figures clearly show that each increment of fertilizer (67 kg of nitrogen per hectare) produces a smaller increment in crop yield as the total amount of applied fertilizer increases.

Inorganic fertilizer can be broadcast on the land or placed in narrow bands underneath or alongside rows of seeds. Fertilizers must be applied carefully; if the concentration of nutrient in the immediate environs of the root is too high, the plant will be unable to take up water, and it will wilt, dry out, and die. Although inorganic fertilizers are usually applied to the soil to be taken up through the roots, the minor nutrient elements are sometimes applied directly to the leaves as a spray. Weak solutions of iron, zinc,

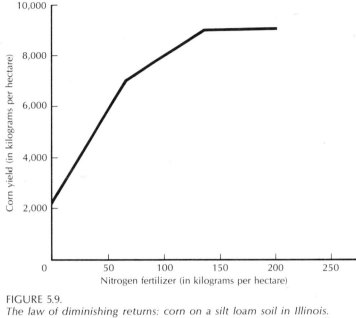

FIGURE 5.9.
The law of diminishing returns: corn on a silt loam soil in Illinois.
(From L. Welch, D. Mulvaney, M. Oldham, L. Boone, and J. Pendleton,
"Corn Yields with Fall, Spring, and Side-Dress Nitrogen," Agronomy
Journal 63, *1971, 119–123, by permission of the American Society*
of Agronomy.)

or copper are commonly used on crops such as pineapple, citrus fruit, or avocado. Such sprays can be used as an emergency treatment if the crops develop certain deficiencies on particular soils. For example, in certain parts of Hawaii that have iron-deficient soils, the pineapple plants are routinely sprayed with a solution of iron sulfate to prevent iron deficiency.

The three plant nutrients used most widely in inorganic fertilizers are nitrogen, phosphorus, and potassium. Large amounts of these elements are removed from the soil when crops are harvested, and they are therefore commonly deficient in agricultural soils. The addition of fertilizer to the soil tends to stimulate the over-all growth of the plant, and hence the production of the crop. However, all crop plants do not respond in the same way to the addition of a given amount of fertilizer to a certain soil. Figure 5.10 shows how the yield of three different crops responded to the addition of phosphorus fertilizer to a particular soil. Even within a given species there can be much variation from strain to strain. Many of the new high-

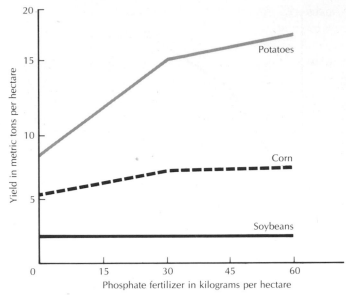

FIGURE 5.10.
Yield responses of three different crops to phosphorous fertilizers on a low phosphorus silt loam soil.

yielding strains of corn, wheat, and rice are characterized by the fact that they respond to added fertilizer with increased growth and increased grain production.

Nitrogen and Crop Production

Nitrogen is perhaps the single most important plant nutrient for agriculture. It is, of course, no more "essential" for plant growth than any of the other essential nutrients; but because large amounts of nitrogen are removed from the soil when crops are harvested, most crop plants will respond to the addition of nitrogen fertilizers by increasing their growth and crop production. Nitrogen is furthermore an important constituent of protein (each amino acid contains at least one nitrogen atom); so the plants must have a supply of nitrogen to make not only their enzymes, but also the seed proteins that constitute an important part of the human diet.

In the soil most of the nitrogen is present in organic matter, from which it is slowly released. Once it is released, it is converted to nitrate

(NO_3^-), and in this form it is normally taken up by most plants. In the plant the nitrate must be transformed into ammonium (NH_4^+) before it can be used to synthesize amino acids. To synthesize amino acids, the plant uses various molecules made from the glucose derived from photosynthesis, and combines them with the ammonium. Research by R. H. Hageman at the University of Illinois has shown that the conversion of nitrate to ammonium may be the limiting process in plant growth and crop production in cereal grains such as corn and wheat. Strains of corn and wheat that are particularly efficient at converting nitrate to ammonium produce large yields and have a high proportion of protein in the grain. The best strains are those which can also reuse the largest proportion of the proteins in the senescing leaves and stalks, and transport the amino acids to the developing seeds. These findings have also led to the selection of strains of corn which are very responsive to large doses of added nitrogen fertilizers. Thus, the high yields of corn and wheat obtained in recent years are dependent on high doses of nitrogen fertilizers.

Soybeans and many other legumes have in addition an entirely different method of obtaining nitrogen. Their root systems are characterized by the presence of numerous small nodules (see Figure 5.11), which are

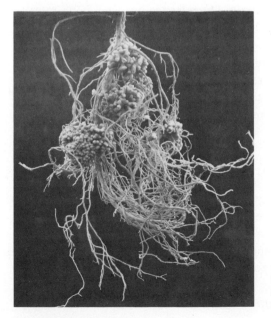

FIGURE 5.11.
Nodules in the roots of a legume.
(Photo courtesy of U.S.D.A.)

filled with bacteria that maintain a symbiotic relationship with the plants. (*Symbiosis* means "living together for mutual benefit"). The plants supply the bacteria with a source of food energy, by providing them with photosynthetic products. The bacteria have the rather unique ability to convert atmospheric nitrogen (N_2) into ammonium, by the process of nitrogen fixation (see pp. 114–117). The products of photosynthesis move from the leaves to the root nodules, and amino acids that are ready to be used by the plants move from the root nodules back to the leaves. Soybeans and peanuts derive about a third of the nitrogen in their protein from the nitrogen-fixing activities of the bacteria in their roots. The rest of the nitrogen is taken up from the soil as nitrate.

One important characteristic of soybeans is that they do not respond to the addition of nitrogen fertilizers to the soil. Even large amounts of nitrogen fertilizers do not result in bigger plants or greater yields, because the nitrogen-fixing bacteria fix less and less nitrogen as the nitrate level in the soil rises. Another important characteristic of symbiotic nitrogen fixation is that it stops during the crucial period when seeds have been set and the synthesis of seed protein is only about half finished.

In Chapter 4, we described the research of Hardy and his co-workers which showed that increased photosynthesis led to increases in soybean protein (see Table 4.1). This occurred because the nitrogen-fixing bacteria were more active when supplied with large amounts of photosynthate. Thus the key to increased crop production in soybeans may be the breeding of strains which are more efficient in photosynthesis rather than ones which respond to nitrogen fertilizer in the soil. A search for the latter has had little success when compared with the high-yielding strains of wheat and rice which form the basis of the green revolution.

NUTRIENT CYCLES

Plant growth depends on energy from the sun and simple chemicals which are taken up from the atmosphere and the soil. Energy constantly enters the biosphere, because the sun continuously provides more energy from its seemingly inexhaustible supply. The same is not true for the minerals and other substances required for life. There is no accessible extraterrestrial source of nitrogen, phosphorus, or oxygen, and life depends on the supplies of these substances now present near the surface of the Earth. If these sup-

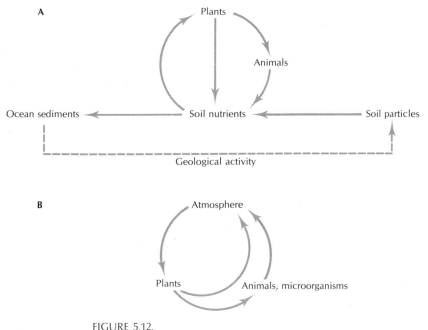

FIGURE 5.12.
Incomplete (A) and complete (B) nutrient cycles.

plies become exhausted, the processes of life will stop. The maintenance of life on Earth, therefore, requires that these substances be recycled. The recycling of carbon dioxide provides an excellent example of this requirement. The photosynthetic activities of green plants would consume all the carbon dioxide in the atmosphere in about five to ten years if the atmospheric reservoir were not being continuously replenished by respiration and burning. Without CO_2 there would be no photosynthesis, and without photosynthesis there would be no source of energy for the heterotrophs. In this section we will discuss the cycles of various nutrients* in more detail. This will allow us to see plant nutrition in a broader context and help us understand how human beings, by means of agriculture, intervene in these cycles.

Nutrient cycles can be classified as either "complete" or "incomplete" (see Figure 5.12). The difference between the two kinds of cycles lies in

---

*The word nutrient will be used here in a broader sense than before, to mean not only those elements released from the inorganic soil particles, but all the other elements necessary for life (oxygen, carbon, nitrogen, etc.).

whether the nutrients will be available in the future for living organisms in general and for plant growth in particular. Complete cycles usually include a gaseous form of the nutrient in the atmosphere. The various activities of living organisms remove nutrients from this atmospheric reservoir and eventually return them to it. The cycles have self-regulating mechanisms, often not dependent on living organisms, which cause the amount of the nutrient in the atmosphere to stay relatively constant. The cycles of carbon, nitrogen, oxygen, and sulfur are complete.

An incomplete or sedimentary cycle is basically a unidirectional transport to the ocean floor of nutrients released from soil particles. Their trip to the ocean is slow, because they may be absorbed by plants as soon as they are released from the soil particles. Subsequently, they may be released from decaying organic matter and reabsorbed by plants many times before they actually reach the ocean as a result of leaching, runoff, erosion, and river-flow. In the ocean they may serve as nutrients for oceanic phytoplankton and other algae, but eventually they will become part of the sediments on the ocean floor and will no longer be available to plants or algae. They may be returned to the land by geological events after millions of years, but obviously they have effectively been removed from present human concern.

Incomplete Nutrient Cycles

Recognition of the importance of the nutrient cycles to the welfare of mankind has generated intensive research on such cycles. Ecologists studying natural terrestrial ecosystems have focused their work on those aspects of an incomplete cycle which occur within a particular system. Such studies involve measuring the amounts of the nutrients in the different components of the system (plants, animals, organic matter, soil solution) as well as the rates at which the nutrients enter and leave the ecosystem. An example of such a study, of the nutrient calcium in a hardwood forest in the northeastern U.S., is shown in Figure 5.13. About one-third of the calcium available for plant growth is already tied up in plant materials (living or dead); the remainder is present in the soil, either in the soil solution or adsorbed on the surfaces of the soil particles. When the forest is burned down to make room for crop plantings, this calcium and other plant nutrients are immediately released into the soil. This release is usually beneficial to the crop, because the cationic nutrients released in this way are bound to the negatively charged soil particles and can be reused by the plants. (Burning also causes some important nutrients to disappear from the ecosystem.

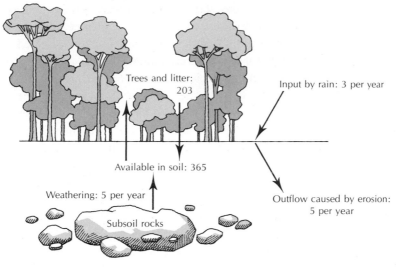

FIGURE 5.13.
The annual calcium budget for a hardwood forest. All figures are in kilo-grams per hectare. (Data from J. Ovington, "Quantitative Ecology and the Woodland Ecocystem Concept," Advances in Ecological Research, *1, 1962, 103–192.)*

Much of the nitrogen in the plants escapes into the atmosphere as a gas.) The study also shows that only a small amount of calcium is lost by runoff or erosion, suggesting that the total economy of the soil is quite stable and that the plants efficiently reabsorb the nutrients which are released by the decomposition of organic matter. Finally, weathering of soil particles adds only 0.8 percent a year to the total calcium; so an exhausted soil will take a long time to recover, as has been known from agricultural practice throughout human history.

One sedimentary cycle of particular interest for agricultural production is that of the element phosphorus. Phosphorus accounts for 0.08 percent of the earth's crust and normally occurs in soil minerals as phosphate. Weathering of the mineral particles releases phosphate ions into the soil solution in three different forms: PO_4^{---}, HPO_4^{--}, and $H_2PO_4^{-}$. Only the last and most acidic of these forms ($H_2PO_4^{-}$) can be taken up by plant roots. In all living organisms, phosphate is a major constituent of the large molecules in the cell nucleus which carry the genetic information. Decomposition of these molecules by the soil microorganisms returns inorganic phosphate to the soil solution. Besides being naturally scarce, phosphate is only sparingly soluble in water. Once the phosphate has been released into the soil solution, it readily forms insoluble compounds with other minerals, and is thus removed from the available soil solution. It is unfortunate that conditions which favor plant growth—the presence of oxygen and a neutral or slightly acidic soil solution—also favor the formation of these insoluble compounds. The phosphate which has been removed from the soil solution in this way can again become available to the plants at a later time. Indeed, the insoluble compounds are slowly dissolved as the plants remove phosphate ions from the soil solution. Since phosphate is an anion, it does not bind to the mineral soil particles, and leaching can remove it from the root environment.

Farmers use phosphate-rich inorganic fertilizers to restore the phosphate removed from the soil when the crops are harvested, and to increase the amount of available phosphate in the soil solution. Phosphate fertilizers are made by heating phosphate-rich rocks with strong acids, such as sulfuric acid. This treatment converts rock phosphate (mainly PO_4^{---}) into "superphosphate" (mainly $H_2PO_4^-$), which is readily taken up by the roots. However, the same processes that cause the phosphate released from the soil particles to form insoluble compounds also cause superphosphate to gradually become insoluble and less readily available. Thus, roughly 80 percent of the fertilizer phosphate added to the soil is transformed into insoluble phosphate compounds.

Phosphate is so sparingly soluble in water that it is often the limiting nutrient in many aquatic ecosystems. Primary productivity in lakes and rivers is dependent on the phosphate concentration in the water. An increase in the phosphate concentration can result in an immediate increase in primary productivity. The increased usage of phosphate in agriculture and in laundry detergents has led to an increase in the phosphate concentration in streams flowing through agricultural and urban areas. This enrichment of the surface waters with plant nutrients, called eutrophication, can lead to water pollution.

Carbon and Oxygen Cycles

Carbon and oxygen are both involved in complete nutrient cycles which are intimately linked to the processes of photosynthesis and respiration. These two processes are complementary: in photosynthesis, CO_2 is taken in and O_2 is released; in respiration, O_2 is taken up and CO_2 is released. The carbon cycle is represented in Figure 5.14. There are three major stores of carbon near the surface of the Earth that are involved in the cycling processes: the CO_2 in the atmosphere; the carbon in the molecules of plants, animals, and dead organic matter; and the CO_2 dissolved in the ocean. Note that there is nearly as much carbon in the living plants as there is in the CO_2 of the atmosphere; by photosynthesis plants annually remove 10 to 15 percent of the atmospheric CO_2 and use it to synthesize organic molecules. Respiration by animals, plants, and especially soil microorganisms returns about as much CO_2 to the atmosphere as is removed by photosynthesis. Thus these two biological processes maintain a constant amount of CO_2 in the atmosphere.

The large reservoir of dissolved CO_2 in the oceans also helps to keep the amount of CO_2 in the air constant. The oceans release some of this CO_2 if the amount of CO_2 in the atmosphere decreases and absorb more CO_2

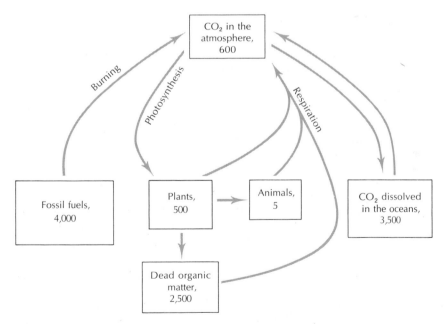

FIGURE 5.14.
Carbon circulation in the biosphere. All quantities are in billions of metric tons. (Data from B. Bolin, "The Carbon Cycle." Copyright © 1970 by Scientific American, Inc. All rights reserved.)

if the amount in the air increases. Several hundred million years ago, large amounts of dead organic matter were transformed into coal and oil, the so-called fossil fuels. These deposits contain about 4,000 billion tons of carbon, which represents 50,000 times the present net annual productivity of the Earth. Since only a small percentage of the Earth's annual net productivity was ever transformed into coal and oil, the accumulation of these fossil fuels obviously required millions of years. The burning of these fossil fuels (about five billion tons each year) has in the past 50 years caused a 10 percent rise in the amount of CO_2 in the atmosphere. This increase would have been much greater if more than half the released CO_2 had not been absorbed by plants and by the oceans. Scientists have speculated that this increase in the CO_2 in the atmosphere may have contributed to faster plant growth, since photosynthesis and plant growth are limited by the amount of CO_2 in the atmosphere (see Chapter 4).

The same processes which recycle carbon also recycle oxygen. Molecular oxygen (O_2) probably appeared in the atmosphere about 1.8 billion years ago as a result of biological activity. Some of the earliest forms of life included photosynthetic organisms living in the oceans. As a result of their activity, oxygen accumulated in the atmosphere, and CO_2 decreased. This oxygen gave rise to ozone (O_3), an atmospheric gas that screened the Earth's surface from a harmful excess of ultraviolet light. This screening probably allowed the evolution of plants, first in the ocean and later on land, and of the heterotrophic organisms which feed on them. The latter, by using O_2 and releasing CO_2, contribute to the rather stable atmospheric composition that exists today.

Nitrogen Cycle

All but one of the inorganic nutrients that plants obtain from the soil are made available to the plants by the weathering of soil particles. The one exception is nitrogen, which is normally taken up from the soil as nitrate (NO_3^-). Soil particles have no nitrogen-containing minerals. The nitrate dissolved in the soil water originally came from nitrogen gas (N_2), which makes up almost 80 percent of the Earth's atmosphere. Since green plants cannot use this atmospheric nitrogen directly they depend on microorganisms to transform it into a form that is usable by plants, principally by means of nitrogen fixation. The entire nitrogen cycle is illustrated in Figure 5.15. Nitrogen normally enters the living world through the process of biological

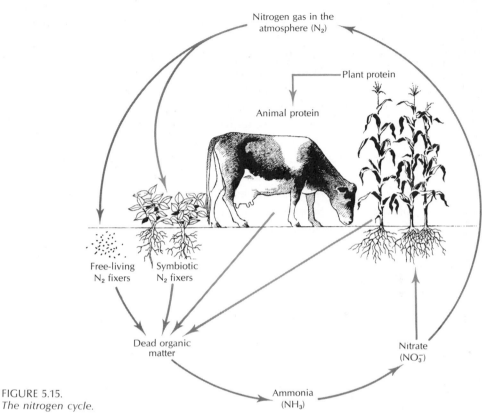

FIGURE 5.15.
The nitrogen cycle.

nitrogen fixation, which converts nitrogen gas to ammonia. Only certain bacteria, blue-green algae, and fungi have the necessary enzymes to fix nitrogen, and they fix an estimated 100 million tons a year. Some of the nitrogen-fixing organisms live in lakes and rivers (algae), and others live in the soil (fungi and bacteria). The most important group of nitrogen fixers for agriculture are those that live within the root systems of certain plants, which include the alder, primitive conifers, and legumes. The leguminous plants (peas, beans, clover, etc.) are the most studied and of the greatest agricultural importance. In the last few years researchers have discovered many new species of plants, including some tropical grasses, capable of symbiotic nitrogen fixation. Natural systems such as forests and grasslands rely heavily on the sustained activity of the nitrogen-fixing organisms in the soil.

Recently Australian scientists discovered a group of New Guinea aborigines who subsist on sweet potatoes as a staple. Their diet provides them with only 10 grams of protein a day. One would expect them to suffer severe protein malnutrition; yet they do not. Indeed, their feces contain as much nitrogen as they take in. How do they survive? It appears that these aborigines may have symbiotic nitrogen-fixing bacteria living in their intestines! Although this possibility has not yet been proved, these bacteria may provide these people with fixed nitrogen in the proper chemical form.

The nitrogen cycle includes three other significant processes involving soil organisms: *ammonification, nitrification,* and *denitrification.* The first two are of special importance, because they make nitrogen available to plants which have no symbiotic nitrogen-fixing bacteria in their root system. The organic matter in soil contains much nitrogen which is not available to plants, because the large molecules that contain the nitrogen cannot enter plant roots. These molecules are broken down by soil microorganisms, the decomposers, in the process of ammonification. The ammonia released into the soil is usually modified before it enters the plants. During the process of nitrification, certain bacteria use the ammonia and secrete nitrite (NO_2^-) into the soil; other bacteria use this nitrite and release nitrate (NO_3^-). It is in this form that nitrogen is usually taken up by plant roots. In a fertile soil, the process of ammonification is slow but nitrification is fast. Thus the plants are supplied with a slow but steady stream of nitrate.

Denitrification completes the nitrogen cycle. Certain soil bacteria use nitrate and release nitrogen gas into the air. They are actually using nitrate as an oxygen source, and so thrive in oxygen-free environments where plants and the other microorganisms involved in the nitrogen cycle cannot grow. Denitrification is quite rapid in soils that have few air spaces or that are waterlogged. On a worldwide scale, nitrogen fixation and denitrification balance each other out, keeping a constant amount of fixed nitrogen in the biosphere.

The nitrogen fertilizers discussed throughout this chapter all contain nitrogen which has been "fixed" (combined with either oxygen or hydrogen) by an industrial process. Until quite recently, the world's principal source of fixed nitrogen to make nitrogen-rich inorganic fertilizers was the deposits of guano, fossilized bird feces, found along the coast of South America.

During the First World War, two German chemists discovered a way to make ammonia by combining nitrogen and hydrogen. The ammonia was converted to nitrate, which was used in the manufacture of explosives. This process, called the Haber-Bosch process, is still the basis for the manufacture of most nitrogen fertilizers. Ammonium salts, nitrates, urea, and ammonia are the most widely used forms of nitrogen fertilizers.

CHAPTER 6 The Origins of Modern Agriculture

In Chapter 5 we examined our knowledge about plants and their interactions with the environment. We gained this knowledge from centuries of farming experience, and, more recently, from systematic scientific experimentation. In this chapter, we begin a description of how human beings can use this knowledge about plants to produce food crops.

In recent years, agricultural scientists have made a concentrated effort to increase food production around the world by breeding crop plants which are genetically superior to the plants heretofore grown (see Chapter 9). This effort has led to a renewed interest in the origins of agriculture and crop domestication, in how crop plants were evolved from their wild ancestors. Plant geneticists are now searching the world to collect seeds from both the wild relatives and the many cultivated races of some of the important modern crop plants. They hope to incorporate some of the desirable genetic characteristics of these wild relatives (for example, resistance to certain diseases) into the modern crop plants. A better understanding of plant domestication and of the relationship between the crop plants and their wild relatives may help plant breeders produce superior varieties of crop plants.

Another reason for the renewed interest in the origins of agriculture and in various "primitive" agricultural systems comes from the recognition that agriculture is part of the natural environment and that agriculture systems operate under the constraints of nature. The success of an agricultural system may depend on how well it can simulate the natural system which it replaces. Thus we need to know more about the natural systems in which the crop plants were domesticated, and about the way in which the agricultural systems gradually replaced the natural ones in many parts of the world.

BEFORE AGRICULTURE

Human beings have been on Earth as a distinct kind of animal for at least two million years and perhaps much longer. Archaeologists believe that this animal first appeared on Earth in Africa as *Australopithecus*. Little is known about the diet of these early ancestors of ours, but it is generally believed that our more recent ancestors were hunters and gatherers of food, and had a varied diet which included both plants and animals. Agriculture, as will be seen, did not become the normal method of procuring food until about 10,000 years ago. One way of inferring the prehistoric diet is to examine our ancestors' buried garbage dumps. These show a preponderance of animal bones—but we must bear in mind that plant parts do not persist in these remains, having been broken down by microorganisms. Some information on ancient people's food habits comes from examining fossilized feces. Botanists have been able to identify the remains of seeds from many plants in these fossils, thus confirming that early people were omnivorous and ate both plants and animals.

Prehistoric people probably experimented with a variety of plant foods, learning by trial and error which were good to eat and which were not. Some of these experiments may have been fatal. Unlike animals, plants cannot run away from their predators, but may resort to "chemical warfare," producing chemicals that make them unpalatable or even poisonous to many animals. For example, some varieties of manioc, a major staple in several tropical countries, contain the poison hydrocyanic acid. The first steps in the preparation of manioc consist of grating the tuberous roots and squeezing out the poisonous juice from the pulp. Many plants contain substances to which people are allergic; others, such as rhubarb, contain toxic acids. Leguminous seeds contain proteins which inhibit the action of human digestive juices. These and other noxious compounds can be inactivated when the plants are cooked. Cooking also increases the nutritional value of many plant foods by making the nutrients more available, and often makes the food more palatable. Thus, cooking may have been important in determining which plants human beings used as food. Archaeological evidence suggests that the controlled use of fire for cooking had been developed by at least 100,000 years ago. This control probably led to an increase in the amount and kinds of plants that human beings ate.

Recent studies suggest that early people did not have to hunt, fish, and search continually just to find enough to eat. They may have had considerable leisure time to make tools, decorate caves, or take part in various rituals and other social activities. Some of these societies of hunter-gatherers have survived into historic times (for example, the Eskimos, the American Indians, the Australian aborigines, the South African bushmen), and for these people food procurement usually takes only a few hours each day. A common misconception is that hunter-gatherers had primarily a nomadic way of life. Those who specialized in hunting migrating herds of large game obviously must have led a nomadic life, moving about in small bands, as they followed these herds. Their material culture and social organization would have been adapted to the exploitation of their principal food source. The use of wild plants for food may have been ancillary in these highly specialized hunting economies. Most hunter-gatherers, however, are thought to have lived a fairly settled life, living in small bands in territories they knew intimately, and moving about less than the specialized hunters. Occupying primarily riverbanks and lakeshores in wooded areas, they probably obtained their food from a wide variety of wild plants, small game, and fish.

THE EMERGENCE OF AGRICULTURE

About 10,000 years ago, a remarkable change occurred in the way people procured food. They domesticated plants and animals, and started practicing agriculture. The hunter became a farmer. This transition has been called the Agricultural Revolution, for it heralded a fundamental change in human beings' material wealth, social organization, and cultural achievements. It also marked a change in how human beings related to their environment. The hunter-gatherer was very much a part of nature, competing with other organisms for the food supply. The farmers started to modify the ecosystem to suit human needs. They interfered with the normal flow of energy in the biosphere and diverted it to products they could eat. They decided which plants grew where, protected useful plants from diseases, and even altered the course of plant evolution, by bringing into being new species that would not have survived without human care.

Human beings have domesticated only about one or two hundred of the thousands of plant species, and of these no more than fifteen now supply most of the human diet. These fifteen can be divided into four groups, as follows:

(1) cereals: rice, wheat, corn, sorghum, barley;
(2) roots and stems: sugar beet, sugar cane, potato, yam, cassava;
(3) legumes: beans, soybean, peanut;
(4) fruits: coconut, banana.

In addition, human beings have domesticated about fifty species of animals, but of these, only the dog, pig, cattle, horse, water buffalo, goat, sheep, and chicken are of great economic importance. We do not know whether many attempts at domestication failed, but current attempts suggest that the list of plants and animals which can be domesticated is by no means exhausted. In recent times, man has domesticated the rubber tree and penicillin-producing molds. Efforts are now being made to domesticate several large African herbivores, such as the eland and the blesbok, because the tropics are not well-suited to herbivores, such as cattle, which have been domesticated in the temperate regions.

The problem of how, where, and when agriculture originated offers an intellectual challenge to botanists, archaeologists, social anthropologists, and geographers. In the past twenty years, scientists from these various disciplines have combined their efforts and now have a fairly clear picture of the geographical origins of agriculture. The evidence indicates that agriculture originated independently and almost simultaneously 6,000 to 9,000 years ago in America, Africa, southwestern Asia, and southeastern Asia. The archaeological approach to the problem of the origin of agriculture is to study the agricultural implements and the plant remains found in various excavations around the world. Modern crop plants are often strikingly different from their primitive ancestors, and a careful examination of the plant remains in the archaeological excavations often reveals gradual changes in the physical characteristics of the plants. The approach of the plant geographers is to study the worldwide distribution of the wild relatives of our crop plants. It was observed long ago that some geographical regions contain many different wild relatives of certain crop plants, whereas others contain none. For example, wheat and maize are now grown all over the world, but the wild relatives of maize are found primarily in southern Mexico and Central America, and the wild relatives of wheat are found mainly in southwestern Asia. This observation led to the hypothesis that the area where the wild relatives of a particular crop plant are found may also be the area where the crop plant originated and was domesticated. This general rule appears to be true for some crop plants, but it does not apply to all of them.

Geneticists approach the problem of the ancestry of domesticated plants by studying the genetic relationships between the domesticated plants and their wild relatives, in order to trace the lines of descent and reconstruct a "family tree."

From integrating all these sources of information, scientists now have a fairly good idea of where most domesticated plants originated (see Figure 6.1). Certain crop plants, such as maize, wheat, or rice, seem to have originated in small, well-defined geographical areas which can be considered their centers of origin. From the centers, they gradually spread into other areas. For example, wheat spread in prehistoric times from southwestern Asia where it originated, into Greece via Turkey, into North Africa via

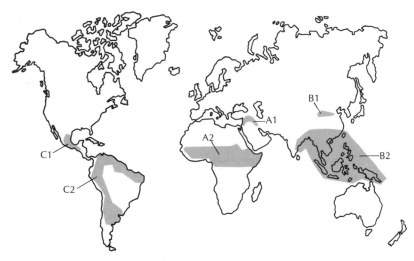

FIGURE 6.1.
Geographical origins of some crop plants.
A1: wheat, rye, pea, bean, lentil.
A2: sorghum, millet, okra, watermelon,
     cotton, yam, banana.
B1: buckwheat, soybean, onion, lettuce,
     eggplant.
B2: banana, taro, coconut, sugarcane, citrus.
C1: corn, bean, squash, sweet potato, chili
     pepper, papaya.
C2: potato, tomato, pumpkin, tobacco,
     peanut, pineapple, lima bean.
(From J. R. Harlan, "Agricultural Origins:
Centers and Non-Centers," Science, 174,
1971, 472. Copyright 1971 by the American
Association for the Advancement of Science.)

Egypt, up the Danube Valley via Turkmenistan, and south into the alluvial valleys of the Euphrates and the Tigris. Many other important crop plants, such as beans, sorghum, cotton, or bananas, appear to have been domesticated throughout very large areas. These crops did not originate in a center, but were probably domesticated by different groups of people living in the large geographical area where the wild ancestors of these crop plants grew. Thus agriculture may not have been "discovered" in only a few places. Rather, it was part of the general change in human beings' relationship to their food sources which occurred nearly 10,000 years ago.

Why did people start plowing the soil, sowing seeds, and cultivating fields? Needless to say, this is a difficult question, and the answer to it is unknown. Some scientists have argued that changes in climate forced people to become farmers. This may have happened in certain areas of Europe where the large hardwood forests provided adequate food to a population of hunters and gatherers. A gradual change in climate may have decreased this food supply and forced the people into agriculture. Others believe that the development of farming was closely linked to the religious rites of primitive peoples. Goats, sheep, and cattle were kept for use in sacrifices. The sowing of seeds may have had its origin in human burials: in many primitive cultures the human body is found buried with seeds and implements necessary for daily life. After an examination of many archaeological sites in southwestern Asia, archaeologist R. J. Braidwood has put forward a plausible hypothesis about why people began farming in that region. He believes that the emergence of agriculture was part of humanity's over-all cultural evolution, and that it occurred as a result of a slowly changing ecological relationship between human beings and the plants and animals they used for food. Agricultural food production developed "as the culmination of the ever-increasing cultural differentiation and specialization of human communities." Perhaps the invention of agriculture was inevitable once people had become thoroughly familiar with the plants and animals which formed their major food source.

Several botanists have stressed the fact that quite a few of our major crop plants are annual plants that grow readily in disturbed soil. Crop plants share this characteristic with weeds. We usually define weeds as unwanted plants that are competing with the plants we do want. But weeds can also be defined as plants which are adapted to take advantage of disturbed or open habitats. Weeds quickly spring up where a disruption of the normal vegetation has left the ground bare. The ancestors of modern crop plants may have been weeds which grew naturally in the disturbed and fertile soil surrounding the semipermanent settlements of humans. Such plants may have sought human beings out just as much as humans sought them out, because of their adaptations and their need for highly fertile soil. This hypothesis of the origin of agriculture has become known as the "rubbish heap" hypothesis, since it assumes that plants with weedy tendencies grew readily in rubbish heaps and other areas where the soil was disturbed and fertile. People may have collected the seeds of the weeds in the same manner that they gathered the seeds of other plants. At first, they may have gathered them from great distances; but the abundance of these plants near human settlements may have increased as seeds were scattered on the ground from carelessness. Thus gathering may have given way to "harvesting." Finally, primitive agriculturalists may have sown seeds in fields or gardens in which the soil had been prepared.

THE DOMESTICATION OF WHEAT AND CORN

One way to gain a better understanding of the process of plant domestication is to study the available evidence for some of the major food plants. Wheat was originally domesticated in a hilly region of southwestern Asia called the "Fertile Crescent" (see Figure 6.2). The area is bordered on one side by the Tigris–Euphrates basin (ancient Mesopotamia) and on the other side by the mountains of Iran, Turkey, Syria, and Jordan. Around 10,000 B.C., this region apparently had a hospitable climate. It was warm, and there was ample rainfall for plant growth. The food supply was abundant: emmer, einkorn,* barley, peas, and lentils grew wild; wild sheep, pigs, goats, and deer were present. The hills were inhabited by hunters and gatherers who had acquired an intimate knowledge of their food sources. Around 10,000 B.C., some of these hunters moved out of the caves and into semipermanent settlements, possibly because their growing population made it increasingly difficult to procure enough food hunting and gathering.

Several of these settlements have now been excavated by archaeologists, and their findings indicate that farming may have begun there. The

---

*Einkorn, a German word meaning "one grain," is a primitive form of wheat with only two rows of kernels in each head. Emmer is another primitive form of wheat which is thought to be a hybrid arising out of a cross between einkorn wheat and wild goat grass (see Figure 6.3). Figure 6.3).

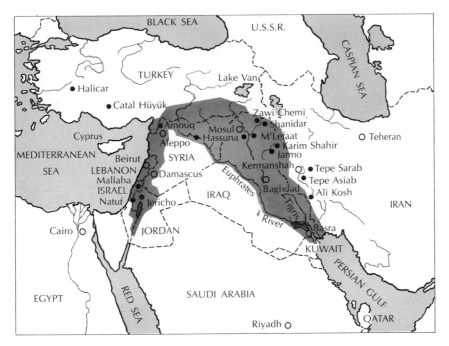

FIGURE 6.2.
The Fertile Crescent in southwestern Asia. The shaded area shows the distribution of emmer and einkorn, two wild varieties of wheat. The solid dots show the location of early permanent settlements excavated by archaeologists. (From C. B. Heiser, Seed to Civilization. W. H. Freeman and Company, Copyright © 1973.)

earliest evidence of agriculture is the presence of sickle blades in deposits dating back some 12,000 years. Pounding stones and mortars for grinding are even older, but they are not distinctly agricultural tools. The presence of these implements suggests that very intensive gathering of grains was going on at the time. Human beings had undoubtedly entered the "harvesting" stage of agricultural development; whether they were also planting grains is difficult to ascertain. The second line of evidence that agriculture originated at that time concerns a change in the animal bones found near the settlements. Bones from goats, deer, and gazelles decrease, whereas those from sheep, especially young sheep, increase. This suggests that there may have been a shift from hunting wild animals to herding sheep. Herded animals are more easily killed than wild ones, and usually it is the young rather than the mature animals that are slaughtered for food. The third finding is that one variety of cultivated barley and two varieties of cultivated wheat have been identified among the plant remains found in the archaeological excavations in the Fertile Crescent. The earliest findings of the two species of cultivated wheat, called emmer and einkorn (see Figure 6.3), were in deposits dated between 7500 and 6750 B.C. The identifications were made from the imprints of grains in baked clay and charred grains found in fire

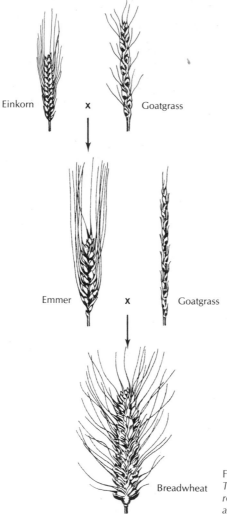

Einkorn   X   Goatgrass

Emmer   X   Goatgrass

Breadwheat

FIGURE 6.3.
The evolution of wheat from its wild relatives. Both einkorn and emmer wheats are found in the Fertile Crescent.

sites. The plants from which these grains came differed from their wild relatives that grew in the same area and were also found among the plant remains in the excavations. This difference indicates that plant domestication had started. Once people started to cultivate plants, harvest grains, and preserve a portion of the crop for planting at a later time, they also selected, probably unconsciously, in favor of certain plant characteristics; so the grains from cultivated plants began to differ from those of the wild ones.

Along with wheat, and later barley, people also domesticated peas, chick-peas, and lentils, legumes which also grew wild in that area. The sites where the first signs of plant domestication were found are believed to have been semipermanent settlements with a population of a few hundred people each. By 5000 B.C., such thriving agricultural communities were found in a wide area stretching from Greece to Afghanistan. The agricultural way of life spread rapidly through Europe and western Asia, and by 1500 B.C. hunting and gathering was practiced only in the northern regions of this area.

The developments taking place in southwestern Asia were not unique; similar changes were occurring in other parts of the world. When Columbus came to the Americas, corn was the most widely cultivated plant, growing from southern Canada to southern South America. It was first domesticated by the Indians, some of whom called it "mays"; this name, in the form "maize", is still used throughout the world except in the U.S. and Canada. The five major varieties of corn known today—dent corn, flint corn, pop-corn, flour corn, and sweet corn—were all cultivated by the Indians. Columbus brought corn back to Europe after his voyages to the New World, but corn never became a major staple in Europe. In the Americas corn has lost its former status as the primary food source. Although corn is still an important staple in several Latin American and African countries, most of the world's corn production is used as livestock feed. Corn has very distinctive botanical features. It is a tall plant which bears "male" flowers at the top in a tassel, and "female" ones in the ears at the side of the stalk. Unlike other cereal grains, the grains of corn are not covered with chaff, and so are more easily accessible to man.

One of the closest relatives of corn is teosinte, a coarse grass that grows wild in Mexico and Guatemala and looks very much like corn. Teosinte is often found as a weed at the edges of the cornfields, and the two plants interbreed to produce fertile hybrids. Several scientists have proposed that teosinte is not only a close relative of corn but also its ancestor. Teosinte, like corn, has very hard grains, and archaeological evidence indicates that the grains of corn and teosinte were roasted to cause them to pop open, exposing the food within.

Archaeological excavations indicate that plant domestication was well under way in Mexico by 5000 B.C. The cultivation of beans, chili peppers, gourds, and squashes may have started as early as 7000 B.C. The excavation of a group of caves near Tehuacan, Mexico, has yielded a clear picture of the agricultural transition in that area. Human beings may have arrived in that area around 10,000 B.C., and were cultivating corn, squash, and avocado by 5000 B.C. The earliest cobs found in these excavations are only half an inch long, and contain kernels covered with chaff, resembling the cobs of modern teosinte. An examination of the plant remains in the different layers in the caves indicates that new domesticated plants were being added continuously. By 2500 B.C., two kinds of beans, cotton, and various fruits were being cultivated. The corn cobs in the different layers became progressively longer, until, at the time of the arrival of the Europeans, cobs were nearly as long as those of modern corn (see Figure 6.4). This provides a striking example of the change of the character of a plant during domestication. Whether human beings consciously selected in favor of larger cobs is not known.

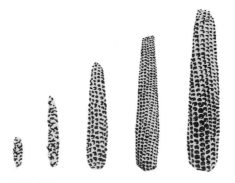

FIGURE 6.4.
Increase in the size of corn between 1500 B.C. (left) and A.D. 1500 (right) at Tehuacan, Mexico. The oldest cob is less than an inch in length.

From Mexico, domesticated corn spread rapidly both northward and southward. It appeared in Peru as early as 2000 B.C. However, by that time agriculture was already well-established in South America, having originated independently in the Peruvian highlands. Domesticated kidney beans and lima beans have been found there in deposits dated around 6000 B.C.

In this discussion of plant domestication, the seed crops, and primarily the cereal grains, have been emphasized. At least one species of cereal and of legume was domesticated by each of the independently emerging agricultural civilizations: wheat and lentils in southwestern Asia; maize and kidney beans in America; sorghum and cowpeas in Africa; and rice and soybeans in southeastern Asia. The seeds of these plants are nutritious to humans and can be conveniently stored. Because of their low water content, they do not spoil easily. The seeds, furthermore, are not only the food, but also the means by which these plants are propagated.

Root crops (fleshy roots and tubers) are an important component of the diet in many countries. The plants which produce them are usually propagated vegetatively rather than by seeds. Many of these plants have actually lost the ability to reproduce by means of seeds, probably because human beings have propagated these plants vegetatively for thousands of years, thereby obviating the need for seed formation. It has been suggested that human cultivation of plants may have started with such vegetatively propagated plants, since such cultivation is simpler than planting seeds. The archaeological record has not provided evidence that would support this suggestion—however, the root crops are grown primarily in the humid tropics, where prehistoric plant materials are much less likely to be preserved than in the much drier areas which have yielded important archaeological information about plant domestication. Root crops, being fleshy plant parts, are also less likely to be preserved than seeds, which contain much less water.

BIOLOGICAL PRINCIPLES OF DOMESTICATION

In the relatively short span of 3,000 to 7,000 years, depending on the crop, human beings markedly altered the characteristics of the domesticated plants. Many of these plants changed more in this period than they probably had in the million years before it. It appears that primitive farmers, knowing nothing of genetics or plant breeding, accomplished much in a short time. They did this by unconsciously altering a natural process, evolution. Indeed, domestication is nothing more than directed evolution.

Evolution is based on two phenomena which can be observed in natural populations: variation and natural selection. Not all individuals of a species are alike; there is much variation. (The nature of this variability, and the way traits are inherited, are discussed in Chapter 9). In a variable population, some individuals are better adapted to the environment, and so produce more offspring, than others. This illustrates the principle of "survival of the fittest," where nature selects the individuals best adapted to reproduce the species. In domestication and plant breeding, people select those individuals that have the characteristics that are wanted. Thus natural selection is replaced by "artificial" selection by human beings. It is not known whether the early farmers consciously selected in favor of certain characteristics, but by their interference with the natural course of events, they may have unconsciously selected in favor of certain traits. Present-day primitive farmers do not—as far as we know—consciously select in favor of certain characteristics when setting aside a portion of one year's harvest for next year's planting. This suggests that selection 10,000 years ago may also have been largely unconscious. A few examples of this unconscious selection procedure are discussed in what follows.

Many wild plants have a seed-dispersal mechanism which ensures that the seeds will be separated from the plant and distributed over as large an area as possible. In many grasses the spikes which bear the grains become brittle when the grains are ripe, and disintegrate when the plant is hit violently (by wind, man, or beast), thereby scattering the seeds. This seed-dispersal mechanism is found among the wild relatives of modern cultivated wheat and was undoubtedly characteristic of its ancestors. Many legumes, on the other hand, have a different seed-dispersal mechanism: when the seeds are mature and dry, the pods suddenly pop open, projecting the seeds in all directions. This happens spontaneously even if the pods are left undisturbed, but it happens more readily if anything touches the pods. These seed-dispersal mechanisms are obviously advantageous to the plant, for they allow it to scatter its offspring over a wide area. But they are a disadvantage to the farmer who is trying to collect the seeds. The farmer would prefer a cereal grain with a tougher spike or a legume with pods that do not pop open. Once people started keeping a portion of the harvest for planting, they modified plant evolution by selecting against seed-dispersal mechanisms. At each successive harvest, they collected a greater proportion of seeds from plants that had defective seed-dispersal mechanisms. As a result, modern wheats have tough spikes and modern legumes do not have pods which pop open. Seed dispersal in these crop plants is entirely dependent on human beings.

A second example of human influence on plant evolution is found in the disappearance of seed-dormancy mechanisms from domesticated plants. Seeds from many wild plants do not germinate as soon as they are shed, but remain dormant for different lengths of time. This is beneficial for the plant, because it minimizes the risk that all the offspring will be wiped out by a spell of bad weather. But for the farmer this trait is a nuisance, for it means that the seeds will germinate throughout a long period of time, thus extending the harvest time. By harvesting a crop at a particular time— for example, autumn—early farmers selected only those plants that germinated in the spring and grew to maturity by the fall. Plants which had germinated later in the season would not have had seeds by harvest time and would not have been selected for planting. As a result, dormancy soon disappeared from crop plants. When a farmer now sows seeds, they all germinate within a relatively short time.

There were three important steps in the domestication process. The important point was not that people planted seeds, but that they (1) moved seeds from their native habitat and planted them in an area to which they were perhaps not as well adapted, (2) removed some of the selection pressures of nature by growing the plants in a cultivated field, and (3) applied artificial selection pressures by selecting for characteristics that would not necessarily have been beneficial for the plants under natural conditions. Moving plants from one area to another can have several important evolutionary consequences. In a new environment, the plant may encounter new wild varieties of the same species or of other species with which it could interbreed. Such hybridizations are believed to have played an important role in the evolution of our modern breadwheats. Movement of the plant from one region to another may also have eliminated free intercrossing between the cultivated plant and the wild parent population. This would have made the fixation of new characteristics, important to man, much easier. Indeed, the fixation of a new genetic characteristic in a small population of cultivated plants is slow if there is continuous cross-fertilization between these plants and a much larger wild population of the same species.

Plants growing in a cultivated field do not have to compete with other species for sunshine, water, or nutrients. As a result, all kinds of individuals can survive which would not have survived under the conditions prevailing in the natural habitat. The removal of the natural selection pressures by man allowed more of the genetic variability in the plant population to be expressed in the field. Human beings then imposed their own selection pressures on this variable population, causing certain characteristics to appear or disappear in a relatively short time.

It is clear that much more needs to be learned about the origins of agriculture before we will fully understand how and why people changed their mode of subsistence from hunting and gathering to farming. But whatever these origins may have been, human beings and their crops are now united in a firm and mutually dependent partnership.

THE AGRICULTURAL REVOLUTION

Humanity's transition from fisher-hunter-gatherer to herder-farmer has been called the agricultural revolution. Isn't revolution too strong a word to describe the domestication of a few plants and animals? After all, revolutions are supposed to cause profound changes in human existence. The agricultural transition can hardly be called a revolution if we consider that it took several thousand years to come to completion; that is, it was not a *sudden* upheaval in human existence. However, it did change the course of history quite radically. The emergence of agriculture is the very foundation on which civilizations rest. The agricultural transition had several important consequences. First, it resulted in an increase in the human population (see Figure 6.5), probably because it was easier to obtain more food, although the food supply was probably not more reliable—nor the food more nutritious. Hunter-gatherers had relied very heavily on a wide variety of very small seeds (especially legumes) for their food supply. The cultivation of cereals—with much larger seeds—simply made it easier to obtain an adequate amount of food. Jack Harlan, an American botanist, has shown that one person with a primitive flint sickle could easily harvest four pounds of the primitive wheat grains in an hour. Thus, a primitive farmer could have harvested in a few weeks more than enough grain to feed a family for a year.

Population growth led to an increase in the number of settlements, but also—and more importantly—to the formation of cities. Great civilizations arose in Asia, Africa, and the Americas, and in all of them the urban population was supported by a large agricultural population. Living together in small groups required people to experiment with new social and political structures. Urbanization also resulted in occupational differentiation. Freed

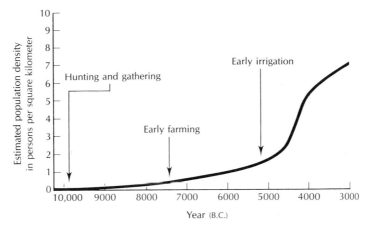

FIGURE 6.5
Increase in population density in Iran during the transition to agri-culture. (From K. V. Flannery, "Origins and ecological effects of early domestication in Iran and the Near East," in P. Ucko and G. Dimbledy, eds., Research Seminar in Archaeology and Related Subjects, Duck-worth, 1969.)

from the chores of producing food, some of the urban people became rulers, priests, soldiers, traders, builders, and artisans. Some of these people directed their efforts toward improving farming, making further increases in pop-ulation possible. One such improvement, irrigation, seems to have had a dramatic effect on the population density in certain areas (see Figure 6.5). The emergence of social stratification was another consequence of the agri-cultural transition. Society now consisted of different classes: an upper class which owned the means of production (the land); a middle class of traders, artisans, and soldiers; and a laboring class of agricultural and other workers.

Archaeologist K. Flannery has suggested that this social stratification was not a result of the success of agriculture (fewer people being needed to produce the necessary food), but rather of the widening gap between the size of the population and the land area on which it was most dependent for its food. He made a study of the rise of agriculture in Iran, and found that 35 percent of the land was suitable for a hunting-gathering type of existence, with the rest of the land being uninhabitable deserts and lands of marginal productivity. The introduction of farming resulted in an increase in the population, even though probably only 10 percent of the area of Iran was suitable for farming. Irrigation boosted population densities even further, although it could only be applied to a very small proportion (less than 1 percent) of the land. Thus more and more people became dependent on less and less land for their food. Those who owned this land became the ruling class. Another consequence of the agricultural transition was that it increased human beings' potential to alter and destroy nature. The spread of agriculture caused natural systems to be replaced by agricultural ones. This made it impossible for people to return to their former means of subsistence even if they had wanted to. Thus, the agricultural transition was truly a revolution which irreversibly changed the course of history.

THE EMERGENCE OF MODERN AGRICULTURE

To measure the rate of agricultural progress in the thousands of years which followed the domestication of the major crop plants is an impossible task. Measured by present-day standards, progress was very slow. The introduction of irrigation, perhaps as early as 5000 B.C. in southwestern Asia, and the invention of such "simple" devices as the plow, the yoke, the wheel, and the waterwheel, were major steps forward toward making food production easier. The agricultural transition set in motion a worldwide population increase, accompanied by a steady expansion of the cultivated area. It is thought that this expansion came about as the early farmers migrated with their crop plants and domesticated animals into areas previously occupied by hunter-gatherers. The spread of the domesticated plants caused them to differentiate into different varieties, each adapted to its own area. It also resulted in the domestication of new plants. For example, the ancestors of our domesticated oat and rye plants are believed to have been weeds that originally grew in wheat fields. When wheat spread into central and northern Europe, the oats and rye became crop plants themselves, because they were much better adapted than wheat to the poor soils and colder climates of the north.

By the year A.D. 1500 the agricultural way of life had spread throughout the world, and hunting-gathering as a mode of subsistence was practiced by only a minority. However, food procurement remained man's major preoccupation. Although some people had been freed from the land, it is generally estimated that two-thirds of all people were engaged in food production. The efficiency of agriculture was low, and one family could not grow much more food than it needed for itself. Contrast this with the situation today, when, according to the FAO, only one person in five is a farmer. Freeing most people from the land has been a major contribution of modern agriculture to society.

Modern agriculture has it roots in the European Renaissance (1400–1600). The voyages of the great explorers and the birth of scientific experimentation took place during this cultural revival of western Europe. The voyages of Columbus and of the other explorers set in motion an exchange of crops, domesticated animals, and farming practices between the different continents. This exchange greatly altered the global distribution of certain species of plants and animals, and increased the earth's capacity for food production. Crops which had been domesticated in one region often found an equally or even more suitable growing area on an entirely different continent. The white potato, originally domesticated in the highlands of Bolivia and Peru, was brought to Europe, and soon became the staple food for millions of people. The reliance on the potato as a staple was so great that two successive crop failures in Ireland in the 1840's led to widespread famine. Although the Irish at that time also grew wheat, they were forced to export it to England; so the disaster was worse than it could have been. By the nineteenth century, wheat had spread from its center of origin to Europe, North Africa, and North America. The western Great Plains of the U.S., with their fertile prairie soil and dry summers, provided an ideal growing environment for wheat and some of the other small cereals. Corn, which the Indians had domesticated, spread over the Americas and was brought to Europe by Columbus. It is now grown in Italy, Spain, the U.S.S.R., Thailand, Kenya, and many other countries. Corn also greatly extended its range within North America. The North American Indians had not domesticated any draught animals, and had been unable to break up the heavy sod of the midwestern prairies. The Europeans, with their horses and oxen, were able to open up these lands for agricultural production. This area, with its hot summers and abundant precipitation, is ideally suited for corn and also for soybeans, which are now a major crop in the U.S., having been introduced from China at the beginning of this century. Rice first spread over Southeast Asia, and more recently into Africa and into North and South America. Rice production is now rapidly increasing, both in Asia and elsewhere. Sorghum, now a major cereal grown in the U.S., came from Africa. Sugar cane spread from Southeast Asia to Central America.

Contact between the different civilizations also spread agricultural practices from one region to another. When Columbus arrived in America, European agriculture was in many ways more advanced than that of the

Indians. The latter, however, used some important techniques not widely practiced by the Europeans. The Indians practiced intercropping—the growing of two or more crops in the same field—and planted seeds individually in rows. The Europeans, on the other hand, practiced crop rotation—growing one crop one year and another one the next on the same field—and spread the seeds by broadcasting them over the land. The Indians intercropped cereals (corn) and legumes (common bean), whereas the Europeans often rotated cereals (wheat, barley, or other small grains) and legumes (clover, for fodder for their animals). Modern farming uses both crop rotation and an elaboration of the Indians' planting method. Crop rotation results in better pest control by not allowing pest populations to build up, and planting seeds in rows allows for easier weed control.

Europe's cultural revival in the fifteenth and sixteenth centuries also resulted in a great proliferation of basic scientific investigation, some of which was soon turned into agricultural technology. A renewed interest in medicine first caused an increase in the publication of "herbals," treatises which described and catalogued plants and listed their medicinal values. The study of plants became a science, and the invention of the microscope in the seventeenth century allowed botanists to examine and describe plant structure in detail. Later botanists, as we saw in earlier chapters, gained extensive knowledge of photosynthesis and plant nutrition. These studies could now be put to use. While studying the mineral nutrition of plants, von Liebig formulated "the law of the minimum," which states that the growth of a plant is limited by the one nutrient which is in shortest supply. An understanding of this basic principle led directly to the manufacture and use of inorganic fertilizers. Knowledge of soil characteristics and of the physiological requirements of plants allowed farmers to manipulate the environment more intelligently to coax the most food from their land. Knowledge of the laws of heredity led to a more rational approach to plant breeding. At the same time, crop production was improved by the use of better farm implements and machines. For example, in 1831 Cyrus McCormick invented the mechanical reaper, which harvests grain as it moves across the field. As a result, one person could harvest much more grain than ever before.

These developments in the last 400 years have enabled human beings to produce food much more efficiently. In the process, however, agriculture has become completely dependent on science and technology. The output of agriculture has greatly increased, but so have the "inputs." Until 500 years ago the inputs were quite simple: they consisted of a portion of last year's crop, some manure, perhaps an ox and a plow, and a hoe. Today, the inputs are provided by a host of agricultural industries virtually unknown 150 years ago. Chemical plants annually produce millions of tons of fertilizers, pesticides, and herbicides. Factories provide a whole inventory of specialized equipment for tilling the soil, applying fertilizers, planting, hoeing, harvesting, and storing the crops. Plant breeders constantly try to obtain better varieties which produce yet more food. Much of this food is not sold fresh to the consumers, but must first be processed in factories. Thus food production in industrialized countries has become a highly complex process.

CHAPTER 7 Modern Agricultural Practice

Population growth and advances in food production have tended to be mutually reinforcing during the last 10,000 years. The enormous population growth which has taken place in the last 75 years has compelled human beings to alter the biosphere extensively in order to meet their food needs. Agriculture has become one of the world's largest enterprises. Crops now replace the Earth's original cover of grass and forest on 1.3 billion hectares. This amounts to 10 percent of the Earth's total land surface, and a much larger fraction of the land capable of supporting vegetation. However, all the potentially arable land has not yet been put to the plow; an estimated 2.6 billion hectares of potentially arable land remain uncultivated.

CROPPING SYSTEMS AND LAND USE

Farming methods vary from the rather "primitive" slash-and-burn agriculture of the tropics to the highly mechanized farming systems of the industrialized countries. But the goals of most farmers are the same: to maximize production per unit of land area, to minimize the year-to-year variations in production, and to prevent the long-term degradation of the productive capacity of the land. Farmers operating in a cash economy have the additional goal of maximizing their profits. The goals can be met in different ways, depending on the climate, the soil type, the available technology, and the food preferences and other social customs of the population. All of these determine which farming system will be used for the production of food.

The system which uses the land least intensively is called *shifting agriculture.* In this system, found primarily in the humid tropics, the land is cleared by burning the trees, and is used for cropping for a few years only. This short period of crop production is followed by a long period of fallow (ten to twenty years), during which no crops are planted and the natural vegetation is allowed to return. Meanwhile, another area of land is cleared, and the whole process starts over. As a result, there is a shift in the cultivated area and the human settlements. Pressures from an expanding population and the need for cash crops can lead to a gradual shortening of the fallow and an extension of the period of farming. Typically, 3, 5, or 10 years of cropping are followed by 3, 5, or 10 years of fallow. Such a farming system is known as *semipermanent cultivation.* It is found primarily in tropical areas where a long fallow is not required to restore the fertility of the soil. In some areas, the land is seeded with a desirable forage crop, and grasses cover the land during the fallow. The next step up in intensifying land usage is the practice of *crop rotation,* in which one year of fallow is included in a three-to-five year cycle of crops. The fallow land is usually planted with a leguminous forage crop, which can be used to feed animals and enriches the soil in nitrogen.

Permanent cultivation is achieved when the occasional fallow is eliminated, and food or cash crops are grown every year. Permanent cultivation is the most common system in many temperate and semitropical regions. It can be carried out on either rain-fed or irrigated land. Many soils in dry areas are quite fertile because their nutrients do not quickly leach out. The introduction of irrigation to such areas can raise crop production considerably. Permanent cultivation does not necessarily mean that the same crop is grown year after year on the same land, for crop rotations are often part of a permanent cultivation system. Even more intense land usage can be achieved by *multiple cropping,* in which more than one crop is grown on the same field in a single year. Multiple cropping is practiced widely in tropical and subtropical zones, where plants can be grown year round, and to a lesser extent in the temperate zones, where the growing season is much shorter. There are two forms of multiple cropping: relay cropping and intercropping. In relay cropping, the seeds of the second crop are planted as soon as the first crop has been harvested. In intercropping, the second crop is sown after the first one has reached maturity but before it is harvested. Additional efficiency of land use is obtained if plants for the second crop are raised in a nursery and then planted between the rows of the first crop.

With such intensive intercropping, the fields are never bare, and four or five crops can be raised each year on a single piece of land. Intercropping is practiced on irrigated land in Taiwan and other parts of southeastern Asia. Taiwanese farmers can grow two crops of rice, a variety of summer crops (melons, soybeans, sweet potatoes, and vegetables), and a variety of winter crops (corn, peas, sweet potatoes, flax, tobacco, and vegetables) on the same field each year.

An entirely different farming system, also found in many regions, is the cultivation of perennial crops either as trees or as shrubs. Most fruits, but also coffee, tea, rubber, cocoa, and other products, are produced in this way. Many of the perennial crops do not provide mankind with food but with a variety of other products, such as spices, beverages, industrial products, and fibers.

INCREASING FOOD PRODUCTION BY INCREASING CULTIVATED AREA

It is impossible to predict accurately what the population of the Earth will be by the year 2000 and how much food the Earth will be producing at that time. Many experts feel, however, that the population will rise by at least another two billion people, and perhaps more if present trends in population growth continue. This means that food production will also have to be increased considerably by that time (perhaps by 50 percent) unless the human race is willing to embark on a conscious policy of allowing people to starve. We pointed out earlier that population growth must be brought under control, but even while mankind attempts to do so, it must also direct its efforts toward increasing food production. This can be done by expanding the cultivated area, and by increasing the amount of food produced on a given area.

For thousands of years agricultural production expanded steadily by expanding the cultivated area. If population pressures caused a greater demand for food, people simply put more land under the plow. The frontiers were pushed back continually as people converted more forests and grasslands to farmlands. This had (and still has) great implications for world politics: nations conquered other nations so that the latter could feed their conquerors. Such colonialism allowed the populations of several European countries to increase far above their own abilities to produce food.

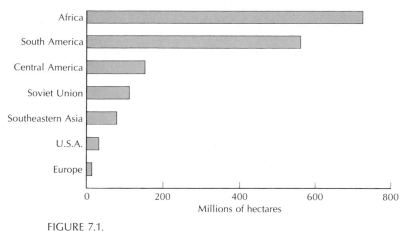

FIGURE 7.1.
Uncultivated arable land in the world. (Data from F.A.O., 1972.)

As the Earth's population continues to increase, there is a serious question whether increasing the cultivated area can feed the world. We now cultivate about 1.3 billion hectares, and about twice as much potentially arable land has not yet been brought under cultivation. Much of this uncultivated land is in Africa, Australia, and South America (see Figure 7.1). These figures are somewhat misleading, however, because much of the uncultivated land is located in tropical areas, where continuous cropping of the type practiced in subtropical and temperate zones has not been successful. However, even if suitable agricultural systems can be found for intensive food production in these areas, the cost of converting this land to agriculture may be prohibitive. Clearing the land, building roads to markets, installing irrigation systems where needed, providing settlers with the essential services, and extending credit to begin farming operations are expensive. Agriculture economists estimate that it costs from $500 to $4,000 depending on the location, to put a hectare of land into cultivation. One cultivated hectare can feed about three people at present levels of agricultural efficiency. Figuring on $2,000 per hectare (an average figure) we can estimate that more than $500 billion would have to be spent to open up new lands just to feed the people who will be added to the world's population during the next decade. Various governments around the world have drawn up plans and allocated money for opening up new lands, but their combined plans and money allocations do not approach 20 percent of this figure for the next decade.

Therefore, excessive costs and the limits of the land will severely hamper future development of additional land for agriculture. Our hopes for increasing the world's food supply must instead depend on increasing the yields of crops and on decreasing the consumption of animal products in industrialized countries.

Agricultural Potential of the Tropics

Most of the unused but potentially arable land of the Earth is situated in the tropics, a region characterized by high rainfall and high temperatures. These characteristics would seem to be ideal for agriculture. Indeed, since the early days of European colonialism, scientists have marveled at the luxuriance of the tropical vegetation and expressed confidence that the application of agricultural technology would transform the area into the bread-basket of the world. That this transformation has not yet occurred has often been ascribed to the cultural and economic "backwardness" of the region. But scientists are now beginning to realize that agricultural production in the tropics is subject to serious constraints, and that the luxuriant tropical vegetation will not be easily replaced by equally luxuriant crops.

Although the tropics have vast areas of unused land, nearly three-fourths of this land contains highly weathered soils (see Table 7.1). The high rainfall and high temperatures in the humid tropics cause soil-forming processes to proceed rapidly, resulting in deep soils which are highly weathered and leached of nutrients. Physically, such soils are ideally suited for plant growth, because they have a thick A horizon and are well aerated. The water from the tropical downpours percolates rapidly into such soils, and cultivation is possible almost immediately after a heavy rain. However, the soil quickly loses this physical structure if it is allowed to dry out when exposed to the hot sun. The soil may become very hard, and in many tropical areas it is used for making bricks. Such red soils, called laterites, have long been thought of as being characteristic of the tropics. But recent surveys have shown that less than 10 percent of tropical soils are laterites. Most of the soils of the jungles have abundant organic matter, but, because high temperatures accelerate microbial decay, there is a high turnover rate of the litter on the forest floor. The high rainfall leaches many of the anions (nitrate, sulfate) and cations (potassium, calcium, magnesium) out of the upper soil layers, making the soil poor in plant nutrients and high in acidity. As a result, phosphate readily combines with the oxides of iron and aluminum (which are abundantly present and account for the red color of some highly weathered soils) to form insoluble complexes.

Table 7.1. Present and potentially arable land in the tropics.[a]

Region	Cultivated (in millions of hectares)	Potentially arable (in millions of hectares)	Percent of potentially arable that has highly weathered soil
Africa	160	600	76
Asia	500	280	39
Americas	300	480	94
Australasia	16	520	31
Total	976	1,880	73

[a]From U.S. President's Science Advisory Committee, *World Food Problem* (1967), vol. II, p. 431.

Tropical soils can support a luxuriant vegetation because the rain forest protects and maintains the soil in a delicate equilibrium. The organic matter that falls from the trees is rapidly decomposed, and the products of this decomposition feed the plants. This continuous cycle of growth and decay relies heavily on a small amount of plant nutrients, but a very rapid turnover. Once the forest has been cleared for agriculture and the trees have been burned, this balance is upset and soil fertility declines rapidly. Burning the trees releases the nutrients contained within them, but these are leached out of the soil within a few years. Removing the trees also exposes the soil to direct sunlight and results in a dramatic increase in soil temperature. This increase causes an even more rapid decomposition of the organic matter, but the nutrients which are released are again quickly leached out of the soil by the heavy rains. Thus it is often difficult to maintain the fertility of these highly weathered soils even if large amounts of inorganic fertilizers are used, because the fertilizers are subjected to the same conditions as the nutrients normally released by the soil particles, and undergo the same fate. The phosphate is fixed into insoluble complexes, and the nitrogen is rapidly converted to nitrate and then leached out. The fertility of such soils can be maintained by use of large amounts of organic matter in addition to the inorganic fertilizers, as was shown by experiments carried out by Belgian scientists in Central Africa (see Table 7.2). Plots of land were cleared, planted with cotton, and treated in four different ways. Nothing was added to the soil in the first treatment; inorganic fertilizers (nitrogen, phosphorus, potassium, calcium, sulfur) were added in the second; a grass mulch was applied in the third; and both grass mulch and fertilizer were added in the fourth treatment. Cotton yields were nearly twice as great if both fertilizers and mulch were used than they were with fertilizers alone.

Table 7.2. Contribution of mulch and fertilizer to maintenance of soil fertility (cotton yield in kilograms per hectare).[a]

	Clean-weeded		Mulched	
	No fertilizer	Fertilized since 1953	No fertilizer	Fertilized since 1953
1947–48	1,032	—	1,127	—
1953–54	200	440	1,117	1,434
1955–56	186	797	1,464	1,977
1956–57	124	706	986	1,344

[a]From F. Jurion and J. Henry, *Can Primitive Farming Be Modernized?* (Congo: Institute for Agricultural Studies, 1969).

The climatic conditions which limit the agricultural potential of tropical soils also affect plant growth directly. We saw earlier (Chapter 4) that the productivity of photosynthesis is reduced by the respiratory activities of plants, and that these losses are especially high when both daytime and night temperatures are high. In a temperate-zone forest, 55 percent of the gross productivity of the plants is lost as respiration; this figure goes up to 75 percent in a tropical rain forest. The importance of this loss for agricultural production is illustrated by experiments carried out by the International Rice Research Institute. Rice was grown in two temperate-zone countries (Japan and Australia) and two tropical countries (the Philippines and Malaysia), and the total production of organic matter as well as the rice yield were measured. The production of organic matter totaled 14.3 tons per hectare in Japan and Australia as against 12.3 tons per hectare in the tropical countries. The average grain yield in Japan and Australia was nearly 80 percent greater than that of the tropical countries (8.9 tons per hectare against 5.0 tons per hectare in the Philippines and Malaysia). These results suggest that climatic conditions may limit the agricultural productivity of the tropics because too much of the gross productivity of the plant is lost during respiration.

The native inhabitants of the humid tropics evolved an agricultural system adapted to their environment. In this system of shifting agriculture, the long period of fallow after a short period of crop production allows the fertility of the soil to recover slowly, as the natural vegetation reestablishes itself during the fallow. The cultivated area shifts from place to place, and eventually comes back to its original site. It is interesting that more than thirty years of agricultural research by Belgian scientists in

Central Africa did not result in the establishment of a system of continuous agricultural cultivation. Instead, the colonial government of the former Belgian Congo finally chose to institutionalize shifting agriculture in the so-called "corridor system." Under this system, every farmer was allocated a piece of land which was divided into seven strips. Each strip in turn was cleared, worked for a few years, and then allowed to return to fallow, and the farming operation moved from one side of the piece of land to the other. Many agricultural researchers have not given up the idea of finding a suitable system of continuous cultivation in the tropics. The International Institute of Tropical Agriculture in Ibadan, Nigeria, is one of the research institutes which continue to look for new ways to increase the agricultural productivity of the tropics.

INCREASING FOOD PRODUCTION BY INCREASING YIELD

Because there is continually less uncultivated land that is suitable for use to increase agricultural production people are increasingly devising methods to obtain more food by increasing the yields of the lands that are already under cultivation. Yield is defined as the amount of food that can be grown on a given unit area of land in a given amount of time, usually a year. Three methods for increasing yield—maximizing plant nutrition, minimizing competition for the food plants by organisms other than human beings, and improving the inherent capabilities of the plants themselves—will be dealt with in the next three chapters of this book.

Increases in yield have come about quite recently, and are the result of an accumulation of basic knowledge of plant physiology and its practical applications. Since the developed countries can afford to do the necessary research and development, they were the first to switch from an agricultural expansion based on increasing the area under cultivation to one based on increases in yield. It has only been during the last few decades that the poor countries have started to apply the new technologies and to become "yield-dependent" regions. Statistics from the F.A.O. illustrate this point (see Table 7.3). In the 1960–1971 period, increases in cultivated area contributed significantly to the total increase in production in underdeveloped regions. In North America, however, the area under cultivation actually shrank, because of the now-terminated governmental practice of paying farmers not to grow crops on tillable acreage in order to keep crop prices up.

Table 7.3. Contributions of increase in area of cultivated land and of increase in yield per unit area of land to total increase in grain production, 1960–1971.[a]

Region	Percent of total increase caused by increase in	
	Area	Yield
Africa	43.3	56.7
Asia	39.0	61.0
China	21.2	78.8
Europe	0.4	99.6
North America	−34.6	134.6
South America	57.4	42.6
World	20.0	80.0

[a]From *State of Food and Agriculture* (F.A.O., 1972), p. 12.

A classic case of a country turning to yield agriculture is Japan. By 1900, this island nation was growing crops, mostly rice, on all of its arable lands. But the population was still growing. The government was reluctant to become dependent on foreign food imports lest a hostile nation cut off food from Japan during an international crisis. Short of lowering the nutritional standard of the people, the only thing to do was to increase the yield of the rice crop. The government mobilized the country's political, social, and scientific resources for the task, and as a result the yield increased dramatically.

This "yield takeoff" has now been repeated for several crops in different regions: corn in the U.S.; wheat in Mexico and southern Asia; rice in the Philippines and Pakistan (see Figure 7.2). These dramatic increases depend on many technologies. Among them are irrigation, mechanization, and fertilizers to improve plant nutrition, pesticides to minimize competition by pests for people's food, and the development of high-yielding strains of crop plants. With a given crop strain, however, the yield takeoff is not infinite. Rather, it tends to level off when the inherent capacity of the plant to produce food is reached. Beyond this point, application of inputs (technologies to maximize nutrition and minimize competition) will not increase the yield. This is the so-called law of diminishing returns.

When farmers first apply technologies to a crop strain, there is an initial rapid rise in yield as the amount of input applied is raised. During this phase, the money spent on the technologies is worthwhile, since it leads

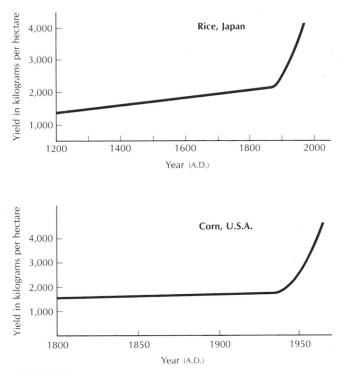

FIGURE 7.2.•
*Two examples of yield takeoffs when modern agricultural tech-
nology is applied to a crop. (Data from U.S.D.A.).*

to a considerably larger output. But once the inherent capacity of the plants
to use the technologies is reached, the great increase in yield slows drastically. At this point, much more input is required to, for example, double the
output. Thus further investment results in diminishing returns. In the developed countries, much more fertilizer, for example, is required to increase
yield than is needed for a comparable increase in the underdeveloped countries, because the former are already at the yield plateau for many crops
(see Chapter 5). A yield plateau will only be reached if all technologies are
maximal. It will do little good to apply adequate fertilizer if the plants that
grow up are all eaten by insect pests. Thus, according to Liebig's "law of
the minimum," a lack of one agricultural technology can be the limit that
prevents maximum food yield from a crop strain.

WATER MANAGEMENT

Conservation and the Water Cycle

Crop plants need large amounts of water to satisfy the demands of transpiration. This process, as was explained in Chapter 5, is essential to plant growth, because it prevents the plant from drying out during photosynthesis. The water available to plants is part of the water cycle (Figure 7.3), which describes the constant circulation of the Earth's water, in liquid form or as water vapor. The driving force of this cycle is solar energy, which causes evaporation of water from land and from the sea. Water returns to the Earth as precipitation. For the Earth as a whole, these two processes, evaporation and precipitation, balance each other. However, over the seas there is more evaporation than precipitation, whereas over lands the reverse is true. Ultimately, the water on land is returned to the oceans via rivers, but its stay on land is often delayed by temporary storage in lakes, ice caps, glaciers, or underground reservoirs. The aim of agricultural water management is either to slow down the loss of water to the oceans (conservation) or to divert water from its path to feed dry areas (irrigation).

Although precipitation ultimately determines the amount of water available to a crop, proper cultivation practices can conserve much of the water before it is lost by runoff or evaporation. Maintaining a soil structure

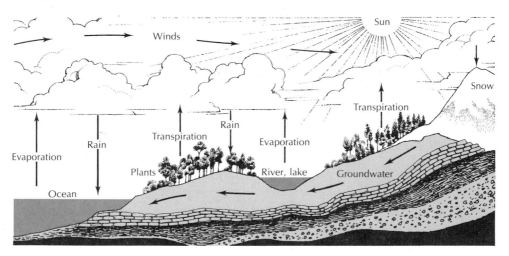

FIGURE 7.3.
The water cycle.

which will allow water to percolate into the soil helps prevent runoff. Recharging of the subsoil with water is an important factor in maintaining high crop production. The presence of a plant cover improves soil structure and water percolation in several ways. When raindrops hit the soil directly, they can easily destroy the fragile soil-particle aggregates, and the air pores between them, at the surface of the soil, making water percolation much more difficult. A plant cover prevents the raindrops from hitting the soil directly, thereby preventing the destruction of the surface structure. The roots of the plants "work" the soil, providing channels through which the water can seep, and the plants contribute organic matter which improves soil structure.

Many farmers throughout the world alternate a food crop with a fodder crop, such as a grass or a legume (clover or alfalfa). The fodder crop is harvested several times during the years, then allowed to grow again, and the entire crop is then plowed back into the soil to provide organic matter. If the fodder crop is a legume, it will also enrich the soil with nitrogen as a result of the activities of nitrogen-fixing bacteria. Failure to manage soil structure leads to excessive water runoff, especially after heavy rains, with a resulting loss of both water that the crop needs and valuable topsoil.

Water loss from the soil can be reduced in several ways. Evaporation can be reduced by leaving the crop residues on the field during the fall and winter. This is especially important in areas where there are dry winds. The crop residues act as a mulch, preventing evaporation from the soil. They also lessen wind erosion by preventing the soil particles from being carried away. If not enough water is available to grow a crop successfully, farmers let the land lie fallow for one or two years. The water which has accumulated in the soil can be used to produce a crop every second or third year. For example, Table 7.4 shows that the water available for plant growth and the resulting wheat yield for a given soil in a rather dry area are much

Table 7.4. Influence of summer fallow in alternate years on available moisture at wheat-seeding time and on yield of wheat.[a]

Treatment	Available water in centimeters	Yield in kilograms per hectare
Wheat after fallow	15.5	4,530
Wheat after wheat crop	6.3	2,530

[a]From V. Thysell, "Conservation and Use of Soil Moisture at Mandon, N.D.," *U.S.D.A. Technical Bulletin*, 617 (1938).

greater after a period of fallow than after a period of crop growth. The practice of letting land lie fallow is of most importance in regions of limited rainfall. Unfortunately, population pressures often place such demands on the food-producing capacity of the land that crops must be grown every year. Then, when rainfall is inadequate, crop yield is drastically reduced, and famine may occur.

Ignorance of the importance of the fallow period and of water-management principles has been a major factor in the famine in West Africa. The Sahelian zone runs along the southern edge of the Sahara desert, and most of the land receives less than 20 inches of rainfall a year. In the southern Sahel, millets and sorghum (two crops with low water requirements) have been grown. When the population of the area was small, the farmers would allow land to lie fallow for 15 years before using it again. However, rapid population growth, combined with the desire of French colonists to use the land for export crops such as peanuts and cotton, put the pressures of intensive agriculture on lands which could not support it. The fallow period in the 1960's was reduced to only one to five years. When annual precipitation slowed to a trickle, starting in 1968, the resulting drought left little land that had stored water from fallow, and famine ensued. The lack of adequate moisture and of organic material to hold the soil together has led to the loss of valuable topsoil, and the Sahara desert is moving southward.

Water may also be stored by construction of physical barriers to its runoff. Fields can be terraced in a contour system to trap rainwater; this method is also valuable in preventing the soil erosion that may accompany runoff (see Figure 7.4). On a larger scale, impounding water by dams to create artificial lakes for water storage has become widespread. Many of these lakes are small, supplying one farm, but others are large projects, such as Lake Mead on the Colorado River in the U.S., which supplies water for several states. Impounded water must be transported by an irrigation system to the fields, but it does provide a reliable and controllable water supply for regions that have inadequate or unreliable precipitation. Therefore it is not surprising that huge dam projects, such as the Aswan Dam in Egypt, have raised hopes for feeding millions of people in areas that are agriculturally marginal because of water inadequacy.

Unfortunately, the great surface areas of such manmade lakes hasten water loss by evaporation. The salt concentration increases, and soon the water is too high in mineral content to be used for irrigation. For the Aswan Dam, the U.N. has estimated that increases in salt and silt will render water

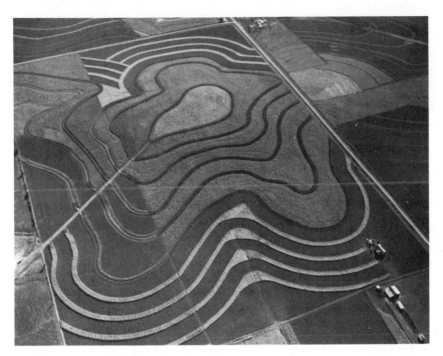

FIGURE 7.4.
Contour terracing to conserve water and prevent soil erosion. The highest part of the farm is at the center of the contour. (Photo courtesy of U.S.D.A.)

from Lake Nasser unsuitable for agriculture within 50 years; this is half of the originally projected lifetime of usefulness for the lake. In the Colorado River in North America, the many dams on the American side have caused the water that arrives in Mexico to be too salty for either farming or drinking.

Irrigation

Irrigation is the bringing in of water to make it available to plants. The water is brought in by pipes or ditches from natural or man-made rivers and lakes. More than 4,000 years ago, the Egyptians irrigated vast areas adjacent to the Nile valley by a combination of dams and canals. A major problem was and continues to be how to raise water from a river valley to fields at a higher elevation. In the developed countries, this can be done by pumps, but people in the poorer areas can afford neither the pumps nor the fuel to run them. As a result, they use more primitive methods, such as the waterwheel. Likewise, the gap between rich and poor is evident in how the irrigation water is distributed: the former use sprinklers; the latter use furrowing by hand or human-powered treadmills.

An increasingly important method of irrigation is the tapping of underground water-storage reservoirs, commonly by the use of water wells. The plain between the Indus and Ganges Rivers supports millions of Indians and Pakistanis. Because of the great water capacity of the rivers, the water reservoir beneath the plain is only ten meters below the surface. Local farmers can tap this great reservoir by driving closed cylindrical shafts into the ground and using small electric pumps to get the water to the surface. These shafts or tubewells have all but replaced the great dam-canal irrigation schemes that had been planned for this region. During the 1950–1965 period, China irrigated in this way about 150 million acres, which were thus opened to agriculture for the first time.

Irrigation provides a water supply that is both reliable and controllable. Plants often vary in their water requirements during the growing season. For example, the high-yielding strains of rice that form the basis of the green revolution are very sensitive to water amounts at two stages of growth. During early growth, if there is too much water, production of additional reproductive shoots (tillers) is greatly reduced, and the grain yield can be reduced as much as 75 percent. Later, during early seed development, inadequate water will lead to inadequate seed production. Therefore, *when* water is applied is as important as how much is applied, and irrigation provides the timing control that is impossible with natural precipitation.

In 1973, the F.A.O. estimated that about 20 percent of the world's 3.5 billion cultivated acres were irrigated.

Desalination

Removal of salts from seawater has been proclaimed by some as the salvation for dry lands. Present methods involve removing the salt electrically (ions have an electric charge) or by means of special membranes. Factories are in operation in the U.S. and in Israel which can produce desalinized water at a reasonable cost to consumers in cities, and these should in the future supply much of the industrial and drinking water for coastal cities. Unfortunately, present and projected costs are too high for agricultural customers, who must in addition pay transportation costs to inland farms. Thus, although desalination may augment man's usable water resources, it will probably not be of direct aid in food production.

SOIL MANAGEMENT

Conservation by Cultivation

Two aims of proper cultivation practices are to conserve soil structure and to maximize the soil's fertility for plant nutrition. One way to maximize the soil's fertility is to insure that the vital layer of topsoil is not eroded away. Earlier, we discussed the importance of a plant cover in maintaining the structure and the stability of the soil, because the roots tend to hold the soil in place. Farming, however, usually removes the natural plant cover completely, leaving the soil bare between rows of plants and after the plants have been harvested. The exposed topsoil can easily be washed away by heavy rains or blown away by the wind. This process, called erosion, is a natural one, and without it most rich agricultural soils would not exist. However, agriculture greatly accelerates the rate of the erosion process, and this may lead to a loss of topsoil. Erosion may be an unavoidable result of crop production, but farmers should do everything in their power to prevent it. The F.A.O. estimates that about a sixth of the land now cultivated on Earth is subject to such rapid erosion that it may well be lost for food production. About 6 million hectares of land are already being lost every year because of erosion.

The presence of forests near farmlands often slows the rate of soil erosion, because the trees act as a windbreak and collect moisture for the entire area. Unfortunately, man's constant need for farmland has led to the destruction of forests adjacent to farmlands, and erosion then eventually ruined the soil for farming. For example, Mediterranean Europe was once dotted with forests and good farmlands. Extensive deforestation has left many areas barren and of little use agriculturally.

Erosion can be prevented by several cultivation practices. In discussing water conservation, we mentioned maintenance of a plant cover and contour terraces as two valuable practices in preventing water runoff; these also prevent the runoff of topsoil that accompanies the water. Some of the erosion caused by wind can be prevented by the planting of rows of trees as windbreaks.

Crop Rotation to Maintain Fertility

Different crops have different nutritional requirements, and the continuous planting of the same crop on a particular piece of land may exhaust the soil much more than the alternation of various crops on the same land. Scientists have suggested that enough nitrogen could be maintained in the soil to support maximal crop production if farmers used a system of crop rotation or multiple cropping with a cereal grain and a legume. The cereal grains normally require much nitrogen fertilizer for maximal yield, whereas the legumes require none, because they (that is, their bacteria) can fix atmospheric nitrogen, which is released into the soil when the organic residues decay. Thus, if both are grown on the same land year after year, the legume may fix and return to the soil enough nitrogen for the growth of the cereal.

Several studies on crop rotation and soil fertility have centered on the soybean-corn system. In normal soybeans, about 25 percent of the plant nitrogen is derived from atmospheric-nitrogen fixation by the symbiotic bacteria in the root nodules. The remaining plant nitrogen derives from nitrates in the soil. It has been found, however, that soybeans do not respond to nitrogen fertilizers, and that increasing the amount of soil nitrogen by fertilizers does not increase the yield of soybeans; indeed, increases in soil nitrate tend to inhibit their natural capacity for nitrogen fixation. Using soybeans and corn in a four-year crop rotation (corn/soybeans/wheat/hay), scientists at the University of Illinois found that adding nitrogen fertilizers to the soil did not improve the yield of either the soybeans or the corn. In addition, corn yields in the rotation system were only slightly below those from corn crops which were not in rotation but which had much nitrogen fertilizer added to their soil (see Table 7.5). Thus it appears that the soybeans can add enough nitrogen to the soil for corn production.

Inorganic Fertilizers

Large amounts of plant nutrients are removed from the soil when crops are harvested. Earlier we discussed three ways in which the fertility of the soil can be restored: by allowing the land to lie fallow for many years; by the addition of organic matter; or by the addition of inorganic fertilizers. The first method is only used in shifting agriculture, but the other two methods are widely used throughout the world. However, when the pressures of a hungry population demand that land be put to immediate use, inorganic fertilizers are employed to maximize the productive capacity of the soil. Because they were (until the mid-1970's) cheap and easy to use, world

Table 7.5. Effect of crop rotation on the need for nitrogen fertilizers.[a]

	Yield in kilograms per hectare	
Yield of	Without nitrogen fertilizer	With nitrogen fertilizer
Corn from		
Corn and soybeans in 2-year rotation	5,800	7,200
Corn and soybeans in 4-year rotation	7,700	7,700
Soybeans from		
Corn and soybeans in 2-year rotation	1,850	1,630
Corn and soybeans in 4-year rotation	1,850	1,850

[a]From W. Walker and L. Miller, "Effects of crop rotation and fertilization on yields," *Illinois Research,* Fall 1966, pp. 3–6.

fertilizer consumption rose from 15 million metric tons in 1950 to 68 million in 1970, according to the F.A.O. Between 1968 and 1973 alone, the increase was 40 percent and was increasing at the rate of 7.5 percent a year. However, price increases caused by the energy shortage (see below) have slowed this rate of increase considerably.

The use of fertilizers throughout the world follows the law of diminishing returns. For certain crops in the developed countries, fertilizer use is extremely heavy because they are near the yield plateau. In the poor countries, fertilizer use had until the mid-1970's, begun an explosive increase, rising (as of 1973) at the rate of 15 percent a year, largely because the newly developed strains of wheat and rice respond with dramatically increased yields to large inputs of fertilizer.

What fertilizers mean for income is shown by a study made in India by the F.A.O. in the late 1960's. Optimal amounts of nitrogen fertilizer generally produced 11 metric tons of grain beyond the normal yield for every ton of fertilizer supplied. At that time, a ton of fertilizer cost $150, and the market value of the extra grain it produced was about $1,200. Even with the recent increases in the price of fertilizers, their value is apparent. Adding fertilizer to the soil tends to stimulate the over-all growth of the plant, and hence seed production will be greater. Often, however, increases in grain yield have not been matched by similar increases in protein yield; although there is often more grain from a fertilized plot of land, the grain is poorer for human nutrition. Recent research on experimental plots indicates that this protein reduction need not occur. When nitrogen fertilizer is applied in the late spring, it promotes protein synthesis later in the life

Table 7.6. The effect of late-spring application of nitrogen fertilizer on wheat yields.[a]

Fertilizer	Grain yield in kilograms per hectare	Grain protein in kilograms per hectare	Percent protein in grain
None	4,700	502	10.0
Applications of 112 kilograms of nitrogen per hectare on:			
April 2	5,760	798	12.9
April 23	5,760	854	13.8
May 9	6,400	974	14.3

[a]From D. Hucklesby, C. Brown, S. Howell, and R. Hageman, "Late-Spring Applications of Nitrogen for Efficient Utilization and Enhanced Production of Grain and Grain Protein of Wheat," *Agronomy Journal*, 63 (1971), 276, by permission of the American Society of Agronomy.

of the plant; so more of these proteins end up in the seeds (see Table 7.6). Delayed application of nitrogen fertilizer can, therefore, result in a more nutritious crop.

When large amounts of inorganic fertilizers are added to the soil, the plants cannot always use all of it. Fertilizers are often added at the time of planting, or well before the plants have an extensive root system. This timing increases the chances that some fertilizer may be washed away, either as runoff or leached into the groundwater. This is especially true for nitrate, a negatively charged ion which does not bind to the negatively charged soil particles. Phosphate is also negatively charged but it is usually rapidly immobilized in the soil because it forms insoluble complexes, which diminishes the risk that it will be washed away.

The accumulation of nitrate in the underground water reservoirs can have two effects. If people use this water for drinking, bacteria living in the human intestinal system can convert the nitrate to nitrite, which inhibits the functioning of the oxygen-carrying pigment hemoglobin, and suffocation results. Few known cases of such poisonings have been reported, but as fertilizer use increases, nitrate levels in the drinking water are being monitored.

A more common effect of fertilizer accumulation in water occurs when nitrate-laden water arrives in a stream or lake. There it may be joined by other pollutants, such as the phosphate-rich waters from municipal sewage plants (most of the phosphates in these waters comes from detergents). In the streams and lakes, these nutrients stimulate the growth of algae in much the same way that fertilizers increase plant growth on land. Some algal "blooms" appear, and when the algae die they are decomposed by bacteria. If there is a large amount of plant material, decomposers will use up much of the oxygen dissolved in the water. As the amount of oxygen in the water decreases, a type of decay that does not require oxygen sets in, and fish that require large amounts of dissolved oxygen in order to breathe soon die, leaving only fish that have lower oxygen requirements (see Figure 7.5). Lake Erie was once filled with trout (a high oxygen requirer), but now contains abundant catfish (a low oxygen requirer). Since catfish are less desirable as food than trout, the food productivity of the lake has thus been

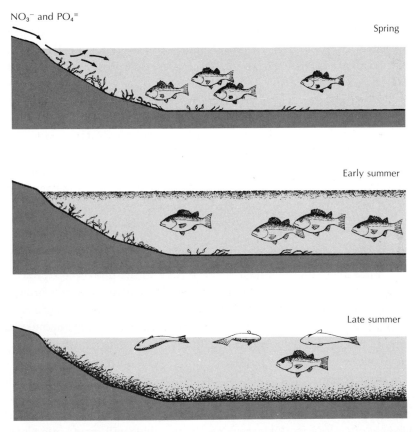

FIGURE 7.5.
Stages in eutrophication of a body of fresh water.

lowered. Similar situations in which fertilizer runoff has caused changes in aquatic systems have been observed in many regions of the world. In the U.N. Stockholm Conference on the Environment in 1973, the combined nations resolved to examine closely this effect of widespread fertilizer use.

MECHANIZATION

As society has become industrialized, there has been a trend to increase the productivity of labor, and even to replace it, with machines. Nowhere has this trend been more evident than in agriculture. Whereas in the colonial period the American farmer produced sufficient food for at most 1.5 other people, today an American farmer can produce enough to feed 50 others. Since 1950, the number of farmers in the U.S. has been halved, but the yield per acre of crops has nearly doubled. Increased use of technological inputs, such as irrigation, fertilizers, and machines, has made possible this difference in productivity per person.

Mechanization helps increase crop production in several ways. Deeper plowing and better soil preparation are possible, and machines can plant seeds at the exact interval needed for maximum growth. Harvesting combines (see Figure 7.6) can quickly pick the crop and mechanically separate out the desired plant parts (seeds, cobs, fruits). Other technological inputs, such as fertilizer, pesticides, and irrigation, can be made much more available by mechanical means. The increases in labor efficiency due to mechanization mean that more land can be worked on by a given labor force. To produce 100 bushels of corn in the U.S., it took 350 man-hours in 1800, 34 man-hours in 1950, 3.5 man-hours in 1960, and less than one man-hour in 1970.

Encouraged by such figures, the F.A.O. in the mid-1960's projected that the number of tractors in the developing countries would grow by 9 percent a year during 1975 to 1985. Two facts have caused this projection to be lowered. The first is the fact of labor and land in the developing countries. If mechanization increases the productivity of agricultural labor, it should allow that labor to be used in other sectors of the economy. In the developed regions, these "other sectors" have traditionally been industries and services. In the mainly agrarian societies typical of the underdeveloped world, both industries and services are too poorly developed to absorb farm laborers put out of work by machines. Such people will crowd into already overcrowded cities, unable to find work. Therefore, to maintain employment (and political stability), the pace of farm mechanization has been reduced,

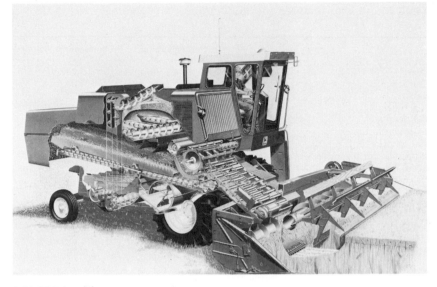

FIGURE 7.6.
The wheat combine. This machine harvests grain, and separates it from chaff and debris by means of a series of mechanical rollers. In the lower part of the machine, the grain is further purified by screens and blown air. Finally, it is put into the storage tank behind the driver. (Photo courtesy of John Deere Co.).

and so have the possible yields. The second fact causing a reduction in the pace of agricultural mechanization is the increased price, and decreased availability, of the fuel needed to run the machines.

AGRICULTURE AND ENERGY

The oil embargo of 1973–1974 showed dramatically the dependence of the technology of the developed countries on energy. High-yield agriculture requires technological inputs, such as irrigation, fertilizers, pesticides, and machines, and these all require energy for their manufacture and use. Indeed, the rise of high-yield agriculture and its export to the developing countries had assumed the existence of unlimited and of cheap forms of energy. Now, neither assumption is true.

Table 7.7. Energy required for production of one acre of corn in the U.S.[a]

Item	Energy required (in thousands of calories)	
	In 1950	In 1970
Labor	10	5
Machinery	250	420
Gasoline	615	797
Nitrogen fertilizer	126	940
Phosphorus fertilizer	15	47
Potassium fertilizer	10	68
Seeds for planting	40	63
Irrigation	23	34
Pesticides	˙2	22
Drying after harvest	30	120
Electricity	54	310
Transportation	30	70
Total input energy	1,205	2,896
Total output energy	3,830	8,164
Corn yield in bushels per acre bu/ac	34	81
Output/input ratio	3.18	2.82

[a]From D. Pimentel, L. Hurd, A. Bellotti, M. Forster, I. Oka, R. Sholes, and R. Whitman, "Food Production and the Energy Crisis," *Science,* 182 (1973), 443–449. Copyright 1973 by the American Association for the Advancement of Science.

D. Pimentel and colleagues have made estimates of the energy requirements and output for corn production (see Table 7.7). From 1950 to 1970, although the yield of corn increased considerably, so did the energy needed to produce that yield, so that the output of energy from the corn seeds per unit of energy needed to produce them actually declined by 10 percent. In an era of cheap and abundant energy, such a situation would be economically feasible. But in 1973–1974, the price of crude oil tripled, and, at times, oil was in limited supply. Although the estimates of the amount of oil remaining for people to use vary, few of them suggest that we have more than 100 years' supply. Clearly, methods must be devised to make agriculture less energy-dependent.

The three major energy inputs for corn production are nitrogen fertilizer, gasoline, and machinery. Much energy is needed to produce nitrogen fertilizer in industrial nitrogen fixation. The Haber process,

$$N_2 \;+\; 3H_2 \;\rightarrow\; 2NH_3$$
(nitrogen plus hydrogen make ammonia),

is by far the most common method for fertilizer production. According to recent U.N. estimates, about 2.3 kilograms of ammonia can be formed from the energy generated by one ton of coal. Several methods of reducing the need for nitrogen have already been mentioned; these include inter-cropping and crop rotation with nitrogen-fixing legumes, such as soybeans. The massive use of organic fertilizers, such as manure, which release nitrate to the soil (albeit slowly) has been advocated by the government of India. In China, use of human and animal wastes as fertilizers has made that country relatively independent of petroleum-based nitrogen fertilizers.

The second and third major energy expenditures for food production are related: gasoline is needed to power machines, and energy is needed for their manufacture. Thus a reduction in mechanization means a reduction in both of these energy requirements. Such a reduction will mean more labor-intensive farming, which will increase employment in some countries, as already mentioned. It would most probably result in a reduction in the stan-dard of living as we now understand it—although many would argue that it would result in an increase in the quality of life. The energy saving is large: Pimentel estimates that, to apply herbicide to an acre of corn, 18,000 calories are needed for a tractor and sprayer, but only 300 calories for a hand sprayer. In the past, labor costs were far greater than the tractor cost as amortized over a long period. However, as fuel costs rise, the cost of mechanical power will equalize with that of human power.

A final way to reduce energy costs in food production is to breed or select crop-plant strains for "low-energy agriculture." The wheat and rice strains which form the basis of the green revolution were bred to produce high yields when given high amounts of energy-requiring technological inputs. Strains can now be bred for such characteristics as a more efficient response to fertilizer, disease resistance, so that pesticides are unnecessary, and a lower moisture content, to eliminate the need for post-harvest drying.

CHAPTER 8

Strategies for Pest Control

In Chapter 7 we discussed the intensive use of agricultural technologies, such as irrigation, fertilizers, and mechanization, to maximize crop yield by maximizing plant nutrition. Many other organisms besides human beings use crop plants as food, or grow in a way that reduces the yield of the crop (see Table 8.1). When the reduction in yield caused by these organisms becomes economically important, they are termed agricultural pests.

AGRICULTURAL PESTS

Weeds

Farmers define weeds as plants which compete with crop plants and diminish crop yield. The conversion of a natural system to an agricultural one usually involves clearing the land, plowing it, and fertilizing it. These conditions are suitable for the growth not only of the crop plants, but also of many other plants which grow readily in fertile, disturbed soil. These plants become weeds. Some of these weeds may have been present in the

Table 8.1. Rice diseases.[a]

Agent	Plant organ attacked	No. of diseases
Virus	leaf	12
Bacteria	leaf	4
Bacteria	grain	3
Fungus	leaf	11
Fungus	stem, root	10
Fungus	seedling	5
Fungus	grain	10
Nematodes	root	11

[a]From S. Ou, *Rice Diseases* (Commonwealth Agricultural Bureau, 1972).

natural system, but their numbers were low because conditions were not particularly favorable for their growth. The same conditions which favor crop growth also favor the growth of the weeds, and as a result they multiply rapidly. Many weeds are not indigenous to the area where they are found. Indeed, the spreading of crop plants from their centers of origin was accompanied by the spread of weeds. Thus, many weeds commonly found in North America originated in Europe, and did not grow in North America in pre-Columbian times.

Many weeds have efficient mechanisms for reproduction and seed dispersal: some produce only a few hundred seeds; others may produce several million. The dandelion is a good example of a weed with an effective seed-dispersal mechanism. Seed-dormancy mechanisms often ensure that not all the weed seeds will germinate immediately; some seeds may remain dormant for several years before germinating. The cocklebur, a broadleaf weed, has prickly burs, each containing two seeds. One seed germinates in the spring following the maturity of the plant, whereas the other seed usually germinates a year later. Many seeds require light for germination, and every time the field is tilled, a new batch of weed seeds will be brought to the surface and will germinate if the conditions are suitable. Some weeds do not reproduce by seeds, but instead have horizontal underground stems which send up aerial shoots at intervals. Examples of this type are quackgrass and johnsongrass, two troublesome weeds of soybean fields.

Weeds diminish crop yield by competing with the crop plants for water, light, CO_2, and nutrients. The actual effect of weeds on a crop may not be to reduce the crop's net productivity, but instead to reduce the proportion of that productivity which goes into the seeds. In an experiment at the University of Illinois, competition between a weed (foxtail) and corn was tested throughout a range of weed densities. The results (in Table 8.2)

Table 8.2. Production of dry matter from corn and foxtail grown in competition.[a]

Foxtail spacing	Foxtail	Corn grain	Cobs	Stalks	Total
1 inch	1,020	3,710	850	2,750	8,330
2 inches	820	3,880	860	2,690	8,250
4 inches	600	4,020	880	2,600	8,100
12 inches	240	4,090	900	2,810	8,040
24 inches	90	4,280	920	2,860	8,150
No foxtail	0	4,430	940	2,940	8,310

[a]From E. Knake and F. Slife, "Competition of Setaria faberii with corn and soybeans," *Weeds*, 10 (1962), 28. All figures are pounds (dry weight) produced per acre.

showed that, although an increase in the density of the weeds did not reduce the total net productivity of the corn plants, their grain production was significantly lowered. Similar results were obtained with a foxtail-soybean experiment. Weeds can also diminish the crop yield by interfering with the harvest. The morning glory, which grows as a vine, can be a troublesome weed if it is allowed to remain in the field until the crop reaches maturity. Its twining stems make harvesting by combine difficult, and this contributes to harvest losses.

It is difficult to estimate the crop losses caused by weeds. If weeds are not controlled, they can reduce yields by 50 to 60 percent. Most farmers make great efforts to reduce weed populations by hand hoeing, mechanical cultivation, or herbicides, but weeds still reduce crop yields in spite of these efforts. Studies by the F.A.O. on the effect of weeds on rice yields in rice paddies showed a 1 to 10 percent reduction in yield because of the weeds.

Insects

From the locust attacks mentioned in the Bible to the cotton-boll weevil of this century, insects have plagued agricultural production. In nature, the population of insects of a particular species is kept in check by the limitation of their food sources and by their natural enemies. Some insects, such as the locust, feed on a broad range of plants, but many insects have very specific food preferences and only feed on certain species of plants. These food preferences are not well understood, but research is underway to isolate the chemical compounds which attract certain insects to certain plants or have the opposite effect, rendering the plants unpalatable or even toxic. Thus in nature many different insects feed on many different plants. In an agricultural system, there are usually fewer plant species, and a few species (the crops) predominate over all the others (the weeds or the plants along the periphery of the field). Insects which feed on crop plants find an abundant food source, carefully cultivated by the farmer, and as a result they can multiply rapidly. Their numbers are kept in check only by their natural enemies or by the farmer's pest-control programs.

Insects can damage crop plants in several ways. Sometimes the damage is caused by the adult insects, such as locusts and grasshoppers, which eat the leaves of the plant, thereby decreasing its ability to perform photo-synthesis. Other insects, such as aphids, suck out sap from the plant-conductive tissue, thus starving the plant organs of nutrients and depriving them of the products of photosynthesis. Much damage is caused by insect

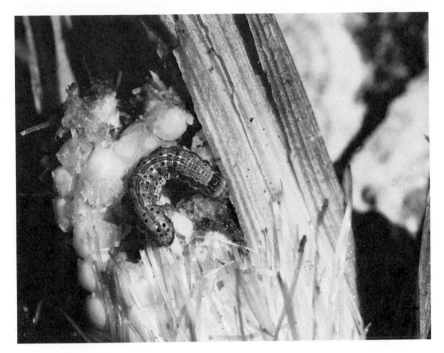

FIGURE 8.1.
The corn earworm, an insect larval pest. (Photo courtesy of U.S.D.A.)

larvae,* an immature form of insects. Some insect larvae live in the soil and feed on young roots, thereby diminishing the plant's ability to take up nutrients; others remain in the foliage or actually tunnel within the plant tissues. Some feed mainly on the stem and leaves, and others, such as the corn earworm (Figure 8.1), eat the seeds. Some larvae, such as the cutworm, live in the soil but come to the surface at night. Cutworms can chew through the stem of a young seedling and cause it to fall over.

Finally, over 200 microbial diseases of plants are transmitted from plant to plant by insects such as leafhoppers. These plant diseases are transmitted like such human diseases as malaria, in which the microbe which causes the disease is transmitted by an insect.

Many insects overwinter either in the soil or in the crop residues which remain on the land. The damage caused by such insects is often magnified

---

*Insect larvae are commonly called "worms" or "grubs," hence the common names cutworm, wireworm, corn earworm, etc.

if the same crop is grown year after year on the same field, since doing so allows the populations of such insects to build up, a problem which can be avoided by crop rotation. However, many insects are fairly mobile, and can easily move from one field to another.

Despite the increasing use of pesticides, insects do considerable damage to crops and depress food production. The F.A.O. estimates that about a sixth of all food crops grown in the world are consumed by insect pests. Even in the developed countries, where insecticides are used heavily, damage by insects is considerable. The U.S.D.A. estimates that 3 percent of the annual U.S. wheat crop is lost to insects. This represents enough grain for two billion loaves of bread, or food for two million people.

Nematodes

In Chapter 5, we mentioned that the soil harbors a large number and variety of nematodes. Most of these tiny eelworms live freely in the soil and feed on microscopic plants and animals. Several hundred species, however, are known to feed on living plants and can cause considerable damage to crops. Many nematodes feed on roots, but some also damage the aerial parts of the plant. Nematodes attack plants with their sharp mouthpiece, which can pierce through the cell wall. They then secrete a saliva-like substance which digests the contents of the plant cell, and they use the nutrients obtained in this way for their own growth. Some nematodes feed only on the surface of the roots, but others live within these plant organs. Nematode infection often causes the roots to die off, and root knots may form (see Figure 8.2). Either condition damages the ability of the plant to take up minerals and water, and the plant may develop mineral-deficiency symptoms. Although nematodes can cause diseases by themselves, the mechanical injury they cause also usually leads to the invasion of the plant by fungi or bacteria. Nematodes play an important role in the spread of viruses. They can transmit certain viruses to healthy plants after feeding on virus-infected plants.

Nematodes, like other disease organisms, are often host-specific. They can attack certain plants, but not others. For example, the soybean-cyst nematode can infect soybeans and other leguminous plants, but does not survive in the soil if cotton or corn are grown on the land. It can severely depress soybean yields, especially if the plants are infected when they are still young. Soybean plants infected with this nematode do not have bacterial nodules on their roots, and are probably incapable of fixing nitrogen. The leaves are yellow, and the growth of the plants is severely stunted.

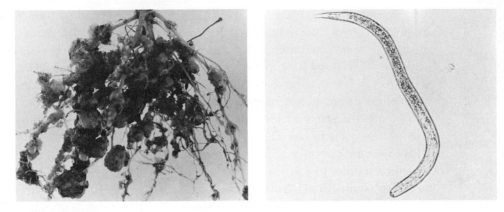

FIGURE 8.2.
The root-knot nematode. Left: Knots on potato roots. Right: The nematode worm. (Photo courtesy of U.S.D.A.).

Fungi

Fungi, commonly called molds, are heterotrophic organisms which derive their food energy from molecules produced by other organisms. Soil decomposers break down complex molecules, and the mycorrhizal fungi, which live in close association with the roots of certain plants, use the photosynthate of the plant directly. Most fungi secrete enzymes in order to digest the complex molecules they use as food. Many fungi can digest the cell walls of living plants, and then use the nutrients contained within the cells for their own growth. Sometimes enough cells are destroyed to cause the appearance of disease symptoms. Most frequently, however, fungi cause diseases because they secrete various substances which affect the normal functioning of the plant. For example, some fungi produce toxins which alter the permeability of the cell membrane, thereby destroying its ability to regulate what goes in and out of the cell. Other fungi produce substances which are similar to the natural plant hormones, causing the plant to lose control over the regulation of its own growth. Many fungi secrete slime which can accumulate in the vascular tissues, thereby preventing the transport of water and causing the plant to wilt and sometimes to die. Such fungi are usually called "wilts." Fungi can attack the roots, leaves, and stem, thereby weakening the plant, but many grow directly on the seeds or fruits, rendering them unfit for human consumption.

Fungi begin their growth from microscopic spores, thousands of which are produced by a mature fungus. They are often carried through the air, and a single spore can produce a new mold, which in turn produces thousands of spores. Many fungi can overwinter in the soil or in plant residues. Sometimes they infect the seeds which the farmer uses for planting. If the mold which causes potato blight is already present in the potatoes used for planting, the plants which grow from these potatoes will be unhealthy and will be unable to reproduce.

In nature, the spread of many fungi is limited by the availability of their food sources (the plants they infect) and by the genetic diversity of their host plants. Fungi are even more host-specific than insects. Spores from a given fungus can infect only a very few species or strains of plants. The natural genetic diversity which exists in any plant species is its best defense against fungal attacks. The selection by plant breeders of certain strains of crop plants, and the resulting elimination of all other strains, greatly reduces the genetic diversity of crop plants. As a result, it becomes more likely that an entire crop will be wiped out by a disease. Once one plant is infected, it is likely that the disease will spread rapidly, because the spores are dispersed by being airborne. Fungal diseases spread not only from plant to plant, but from field to field and from state to state.

Two fungus diseases of importance to argiculture are wheat rust and rice blast. Wheat rust forms characteristic orange streaks on the leaves and stems of wheat plants which it infects. The diseased plants usually produce fewer seeds than normal, with the grain being smaller and of inferior milling quality (see Figure 8.3). Losses from this disease vary from year to year, but in the more severe epidemics the wheat crop has been reduced by a fourth. Rice blast, a fungus disease of leaves, was recorded as far back as the Chinese Ming Dynasty in 1637 as a serious agricultural pest and is now widespread in Asia. The blast kills young plants, and in older plants its effects are, like those of wheat rust, often severe enough to reduce yield. Unfortunately, rice blast thrives on plants grown in nitrogen-rich soils. The blast generally reduces by 20 percent the yield increase that nitrogen fertilizers induce in rice.

Bacteria and Viruses

Some bacteria, such as those that cause decay of organic matter, transform nitrogen and sulfur compounds in the soil, or fix nitrogen, playing a vital role in plant growth and crop production. However, several bacterial

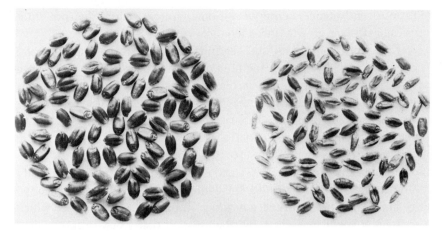

FIGURE 8.3.
Kernels from healthy (left) and rust-infected (right) wheat plants. (Photo courtesy of U.S.D.A.).

species are harmful to plants. Because they are microscopic in size, bacteria can enter the plant directly through wounds or natural openings. Once inside the plant, they multiply rapidly by secreting substances that dissolve the plant's cell walls and then living on the cell contents. Fire blight, a disease that often destroys pear trees before they can bear fruit, is caused in this manner. Another bacterium induces the formation of crown galls, swellings resembling tumors at the basal regions of the stems of many plants. These can be very damaging to the growth of young plants. In general, however, bacterial diseases cause less crop loss than fungal diseases.

Viruses are so small that they can only be seen with the most powerful microscopes. All viruses are parasitic; they can only live and reproduce in other cells, whether plant, animal, or microbial. More than half the known viruses attack plants, causing a variety of diseases. One kind of virus may infect one or more plant species, and one plant species may be attacked by one or many different kinds of viruses. They usually enter the plants through wounds or natural openings. Once inside the plant, they start to multiply, killing the cells in which they are multiplying. They gradually spread from cell to cell, and eventually may infect the entire plant. Virus-infected plants usually have yellow spots or streaks on their leaves, indicating that the leaf cells have died. This reduces the capacity of the plants for photosynthesis and consequently reduces crop yield. Some viruses, such as the corn stunt virus, inhibit plant growth and, therefore, yield.

Like other plant pests, such as fungi, viruses are host-specific, and when the genetic diversity of the host plants is reduced, the chances of a rapidly spreading epidemic are increased. This was dramatically demonstrated in 1971 in the rice crop of the Philippines. In the 1960's, this country reduced the genetic diversity of its rice crop by a massive introduction of the new, high-yielding rice strain IR-8 (see next chapter for a discussion of this strain). This strain was susceptible to the leafhopper-spread virus disease called tungro. In the 1971 crop year, a tungro epidemic literally devastated the rice crop, turning the Philippines from a rice exporter to a rice importer. Since that time, a new rice strain has been developed which is resistant to the tungro virus, but the prospect that a new, virulent virus strain will evolve in the near future remains.

CHEMICAL CONTROL

Contrary to popular opinion, chemicals have been used for hundreds of years to control "pests." Marco Polo introduced pyrethrum into Europe after learning of its use by farmers in the Far East. Pyrethrum is an insecticide present in the flowers of certain kinds of chrysanthemums. By the early 1900's, rotenone, pyrethrum, nicotine, kerosene, and compounds of sulfur, lead, arsenic, and mercury were in common use. However, large-scale spraying of crops was not carried out until after the Second World War. Until that time people used primarily natural compounds extracted from a variety of plants, or simple inorganic chemicals. A significant breakthrough in chemical pest control occurred during the Second World War, when the herbicide, 2,4–D was first manufactured and the insecticidal properties of DDT were discovered. The early successes of these chemicals led to a search for more and better pesticides, and at first agriculturalists were so preoccupied with the effectiveness of these chemicals that little thought was given to what might eventually happen because of the increasing volume and number of pesticides released into the environment. The controversial book *Silent Spring,* written by the American biologist and science writer Rachel Carson and published in 1962, first awakened public opinion to the effects that pesticides were having on the environment. Although these chemicals have saved millions from death by disease or by starvation, scientists now recognize that people have been overenthusiastic in using chemicals to eliminate pests, and that a more sophisticated approach to pest control is needed. Chemicals will continue to be used, however, until other methods of pest control have been devised.

Herbicides

Herbicides are chemicals which kill plants. Some herbicides kill all plants, but the herbicides which are of greatest agricultural use only kill certain plants or certain classes of plants. The most useful herbicides are those which have the greatest selectivity (see Table 8.3). Farmers want herbicides which do not affect the crop plants, but are effective against one or more species of troublesome weeds.

Two of the most commonly used herbicides, 2,4-D (2,4-dichloro-phenoxyacetic acid) and 2,4,5-T (2,4,5-trichlorophenoxyacetic acid), have chemical structures which resemble the plant hormone auxin. When applied at low doses, these herbicides selectively kill broadleaved plants without affecting grasses. They can therefore be used to kill a variety of weeds in fields of corn, wheat, rice, or sorghum. These herbicides are normally sprayed as a fine mist onto the plants, and are then taken up by the leaves and transported throughout the plant. They affect the plants by disturbing normal hormonal control mechanisms, thereby causing aberrant growth. These herbicides are most effective when applied to seedlings or young plants, causing their stems to bend and the tissues to swell and burst. This permits other disease agents, such as bacteria and fungi, to invade, infect, and kill the weeds. The physiological reasons for the selectivity of herbicides are not clearly understood. Plants differ in their abilities to take up herbicides through the leaf surface, to translocate them once they are inside the plant, and, most importantly, to metabolize them. A plant which can destroy a herbicide as soon as it enters the cells is usually not affected by it.

In addition to selectivity, the auxin-like herbicides have the added advantages of low volatility and low persistence. Volatility is the tendency of a liquid to form a gas. Low volatility is desirable for pesticides so that the winds will not carry the herbicide to a nearby, susceptible crop (for example, tomatoes are very susceptible to many commonly used herbicides). Low persistence is also important: if the field has a cereal-legume rotation, residual 2,4-D in the soil from the cereal crop could harm the legume if enough of it is taken up by the plants. Several studies have shown that 2,4-D

Table 8.3. Uses and effects of some common herbicides.

Name	Applied	Effect
Atrazine	By working into the soil to control broadleaf and grassy weeds in fields of corn, sorghum, sugarcane	Inhibits photosynthesis
Barban	As a foliar spray to young weeds, especially wild oats, in fields of wheat, soybeans, peas	Inhibits cell division
Bromoxyquil	As foliar spray to broadleaf weeds in fields of wheat, barley, legumes, sorghum	Inhibits photosynthesis
Cacodylic acid	As foliar spray to defoliate cotton, trees, weeds of citrus	General poison
Chloramben	As granules to soil to control broadleaf weeds of corn, soybeans, beans	Inhibits root development
Dalapon	As foliar spray to grassy weeds in fields of sugarcane, corn, citrus	Inhibits growth
Dinoseb	As foliar spray to seedling weeds in most cereal crops	Inhibits respiration
Paraquat	As contact spray for weed control during establishment of cereal crops	Wilting and dessication
Thiocarbamate	As granules to soil to control weeds in corn and vegetable fields	Inhibits seed germination
2,4-D and 2,4,5-T	As spray to broadleaf weeds	Loss of control of normal growth processes

disappeared within days after its application to a crop, and that 2,4,5-T lingered only a few weeks. Breakdown was caused both by the plants and by the soil microorganisms. The breakdown products (various chlorinated hydrocarbons) may remain in the soil for a much longer time, however, and their effects on plants, animals, and microorganisms are not yet known. Some herbicides, such as pichloram and simazine, can remain in the soil for more than a year. Most desirable are those herbicides which can be easily broken down, by the plants or in the soil, into products which can enter the normal metabolism of the cell. Society's recent concern with the protection of the environment is causing the chemical companies to search for such herbicides.

Because of their desirable properties, herbicides are widely and successfully used to control weeds. Many crops double their yield when these pesticides are used. A second valuable agricultural use for these chemicals has been in the improvement of rangelands. Spraying such lands with 2,4,5-T selectively kills the shrubs, thereby favoring the growth of grasses. These herbicides can also be used to clear forests preparatory to the conversion of the land to farming. When applied to trees, the auxin-like herbicides induce leaf-fall, because they cause the plants to start producing ethylene, the hormone which normally regulates the falling of the leaves. Large areas can easily be defoliated, and the trees used as lumber or fuel.

Nearly 100,000 tons of auxin-like herbicides were used from 1965 to 1971 by the U.S. armed forces to defoliate the trees of large areas of Vietnam, in order to uncover their adversaries' camps. According to a study published by the U.S. National Academy of Sciences in 1974, spraying resulted in the loss of 15 to 20 percent of the commercial timber and up to 30 percent of the mangrove forests of South Vietnam. In some areas, spraying was so complete that there were no trees left to produce seeds, and it will take more than a century for the forest to begin to recover. Herbicide spraying of field crops usually destroyed the crops for only the growing season during which spraying occurred. An important conclusion of the study was that no evidence was found for the direct harm to humans by the herbicides that had been suspected. The reported increase in stillbirths and the births of deformed babies in the most heavily sprayed areas of Vietnam was probably caused by the trace amounts of dioxin present in the herbicide mixtures. This contaminant can be eliminated if other manufacturing processes are used. The Vietnam episode points out, however, that continued watchfulness is necessary if people continue to dump vast quantities of unusual chemicals into the environment.

Fungicides

Fungicides are chemicals which kill fungi. They can be applied as "dusts" to growing crops or as a coating on the seeds before they are planted. Generally fungicides must be present on the plant before fungal spores land on that plant in order to be effective, for they act by preventing spore germination and the initial growth of the fungus. Therefore, as new plant organs form, the crop must be redusted to coat these new organs with fungicide. This need for reapplication can make use of fungicides quite expensive.

The most widely used fungicides are relatively simple compounds containing copper, sulfur, or mercury. Applied to cereal crops, they selectively prevent such diseases as wheat rust and rice blast. However, because these dusts are toxic to man, crops must be thoroughly washed before marketing to remove any trace of the fungicide.

Insecticides

Since the insecticidal properties of DDT were discovered during the Second World War, synthetic insecticides have played a major role in saving millions of human lives. By killing insects that carry human disease agents, such as those that cause malaria, these pesticides have considerably lowered the number of deaths caused by these diseases. Insecticides have also been a major input for agricultural technology, and the F.A.O. estimates that, by 1973, world use of them was growing at the rate of 13 percent per year.

Most agricultural insecticides fall into two categories, according to their chemical structure: chlorinated hydrocarbons (such as DDT) and organophosphates (such as malathion). Both are usually sprayed on the crop plants and are absorbed into the plant. When the insect pest starts to feed on the plant, it ingests the pesticide and is killed. It may also absorb the poison from the plant surface. Because chlorinated hydrocarbons are not easily degraded, multiple applications are not necessary, and one spraying will often protect the crop for the entire growing season. Both types of insecticides interfere with the normal functioning of the nervous system of the insects, causing convulsions, paralysis, and death, but do not harm the plants.

When DDT was first introduced, it was thought to affect insects rather specifically and to be without effect on other animals unless ingested in large doses. However, DDT becomes concentrated in the animals which are at the top of the food chain, and is now present in several species of animals in quite high concentrations. When DDT is sprayed on a field, much of the insecticide misses the intended target (the leaves of the plants) and either settles on the soil or is carried away by the wind to nearby fields, lakes, and forests. DDT and other chlorinated hydrocarbons are volatile chemicals which move through the air, either as gases or attached to water droplets or dust particles. The net result is that DDT is now distributed all over the Earth and is present in all natural waters.

Chlorinated hydrocarbons have two properties which cause them to accumulate in the organisms at the top of the food chain. They are much more soluble in fatty tissues than in water, and they are not readily broken down. As a result, they are neither excreted nor metabolized once they have been taken up into the body. They continue to accumulate in the body if the food source is contaminated with DDT. Thus, the concentration of DDT in the tissues of different organisms increases as it moves up the trophic levels of the food chain. Several studies have shown that the DDT content of plankton is 250 times greater than that of the lake water in which the plankton live. The small fish which feed on the plankton have 10 to 50 times greater concentrations of DDT in their tissues, and the larger fish and the aquatic birds which feed on the small fish have twenty times again as much. Thus the concentration in their tissues is 100,000 times as great as that in the lake water. These high concentrations of DDT have definite biochemical effects: the pesticide interferes with the calcium metabolism of some birds, resulting in fragile eggshells and reproductive failure, and in salmon it affects the nervous system. Although long-term effects on humans have not been studied, the known environmental side effects of DDT led to a severe restriction of its use in the U.S. in 1972 and its replacement by the nonpersistent organophosphates. The latter, however, are more expensive and somewhat less effective than the chlorinated hydrocarbons. These factors have led the F.A.O. to conclude that, for now, DDT should continue to be used in the underdeveloped regions until effective alternatives are readily available.

When an insecticide is first introduced, it is usually very effective, killing off a high proportion of the insect pests. Most insecticides are not specific for insect pests, however, and kill other insects as well. Beneficial insects which prey on the pests are killed along with the pests. Because of inherent biological variation, some individuals of the pest population may have physiological mechanisms which make them resistant to the insecticide. Since most of their natural enemies have been killed by the pesticide, these resistant individuals, along with others coming in from adjoining areas which have not been sprayed, will multiply rapidly, thereby necessitating another application of pesticide. With time the proportion of resistant individuals in the population increases, until they are all resistant to the pesticide.

The introduction of DDT in the Peruvian cotton fields in the late 1940's caused a dramatic increase in yields. However, each year greater amounts of DDT and other pesticides had to be used as more and more insect pests became resistant. Finally, the resistant pests decimated the cotton crops, and the farmers were forced to abandon use of the pesticides and return to more traditional methods of pest control. This story has been repeated again and again, and the numbers of insect species now resistant to insecticides continue to grow. Nevertheless, for the present, insecticides in particular and pesticides in general provide one of the most effective methods of pest control in agriculture.

BIOLOGICAL CONTROL

Control by Cultivation

Good agricultural practices and timely cultivation are among the cheapest and most effective methods of pest control. When discussing various kinds of pests, we noted that many of them thrive only on specific plants or groups of plants. Populations of such pests will tend to build up if the same crop is planted year after year on the same field. Thus crop rotation is one of the best ways to insure that pest populations will not build up to harmful levels. It is probably the most widely used method of pest control. Crop rotation also controls weeds, because different crops require different agricultural practices, thereby decreasing the chances that weed populations will build up. Recent experiments have shown that intercropping also reduces pest problems. When corn and peanuts were grown together in the same field, damage from the cornborer was reduced by 80 percent. The biological reasons for this reduction in pest infestation are not yet understood, but it is possible that the peanuts harbor organisms which prey on the corn borer. Hoeing is undoubtedly the oldest method of weed control, and it is still widely used not only in the developing countries but also in the technologically advanced countries. Farmers normally work their fields, before planting crop seeds, to kill the weeds which have germinated. This procedure brings to the surface another crop of weed seeds, which will germinate at about the same time as the crop seeds. Thus the field will have to be hoed again to kill these weeds. It is important to hoe when the weeds are still small, since mechanical hoeing does not kill the plants directly, but simply breaks up the soil, partially dislodging the root system. The small weed seedlings lose part or all of their capacity to take up water, and quickly dry out on bright and sunny days. Perennial weeds, such as thistles, or various grasses with underground runners, cannot be dealt with so easily, and must be treated before the crop is planted. Although weeds do not start competing with crop plants for water, nutrients, and sunlight until they are several weeks old, it is more difficult to kill them once they have taken hold.

Another important way to suppress weed growth is by increasing plant density. Decreasing the distance between rows of soybeans from 40 inches to 20 inches allowed the soybean canopy to cover the interrow area in only 47 days instead of 67. Once the canopy is closed and the interrow area is shaded, weeds cannot establish themselves. Thin stands of crop plants generally favor a heavy population of weeds; here intercropping may reduce weeds. Recent experiments have shown that corn yields increased by 20 percent when mung beans were grown with the corn, because the beans suppressed weed growth and provided less competition for the corn than did the weeds.

Breeding Disease-Resistant Plants

Just as insect strains can arise that are resistant to insecticides, so can plant strains arise that are resistant to pests. The most important source for disease-resistant crop strains are the relatives of modern crop plants which grow wild in nature, because these plants must be disease-resistant in order to survive. The resistance characteristic can be bred into crop strains (see next chapter). Unfortunately, new pest strains can arise which can infect the resistant crop plants, and so the search for resistant plants is never finished. Pests evolve in parallel with their hosts, and a given pest-resistant strain of plant seldom remains resistant for more than a decade. There are now many pest-resistant strains of crop plants, but a major effort in plant breeding has been to develop pest-resistant strains of the three important cereal grains: corn, wheat, and rice.

In corn, a characteristic termed "T-cytoplasm" was bred into the crop because it makes the male part of the corn plants sterile, thereby re-

Table 8.4. Development of rice strains that are resistant to pests.[a]

	Diseases					Insects		
Strain	Blast	Blight	Leaf streak	Grassy stunt	Tungro	Green leafhopper	Brown hopper	Stem borer
IR-8 (1966)	MR	S	S	S	S	R	S	MS
IR-5 (1967)	S	S	MS	S	S	R	S	S
IR-20 (1969)	MR	R	MR	S	R	R	S	MS
IR-22 (1969)	S	R	MS	S	S	S	S	S
IR-24 (1971)	S	S	MR	S	MR	R	S	S
IR-26 (1973)	MR	R	MR	MR	R	R	R	MR

[a]From *Research Highlights* (I.R.R.I., 1973), p. 11. Key to table entries: S, susceptible; R, resistant; MR, moderately resistant; MS, moderately susceptible.

ducing the cost of producing hybrid seed corn for the farmers. However, plants which have this "T-cytoplasm"—and nearly all corn plants did until 1971—are particularly susceptible to the fungus which causes southern leaf blight. This susceptibility, coupled with environmental conditions favoring the spread of this disease, resulted in a serious epidemic of blight in 1971 which lowered corn production in the U.S. by 10 to 15 percent. Recently characteristics have been found in certain strains of corn which confer blight resistance, and these are now being bred into the corn strains in use. This incident clearly illustrates the dangers inherent in the lack of genetic heterogeneity. If all the corn plants have similar genetic characteristics, they will all be susceptible to the same diseases, and epidemics may devastate the crops in very large areas. Plant breeders have managed to keep wheat resistant to rust for over 50 years by continuously developing new rust-resistant varieties. At the International Rice Research Institute in the Philippines, rice varieties that are resistant to a broader spectrum of diseases are being continually developed (see Table 8.4), and a strain fully resistant to tungro virus was announced in 1973.

Control by Biological Methods

The use of pesticides to control crop pests has often been quite successful, but there are many problems with their specificity, persistence in the environment, side effects, and costs. Some insects are now resistant to the most potent pesticides, and society is beginning to wonder whether the benefits of chemical pest control outweigh the disadvantages. Scientists are therefore intensifying research into methods of biological control, that is, using nature itself to combat pests. As knowledge of the biology of the pests increases, it is sometimes possible to create environments conducive to crop growth but inhospitable to the pests. For example, many pests spend only part of their life feeding on crops, the remainder being spent on an entirely different host plant. Therefore, elimination of this other host plant can mean elimination of the pest. The fungus that causes wheat rust uses the common barberry plant as a host for part of the year. Cutting down these plants has considerably reduced wheat losses due to rust. This method of control has also been successful with several insect pests, and should become increasingly important as research on the life histories of pests proceeds.

Knowledge of insect biochemistry has permitted the development of highly specific insecticides and attractants. Insects produce hormones which regulate their growth and development, and these hormones usually act at one stage in the insect's life cycle. If a solution containing a few parts per million of the hormone is sprayed on the insects at another developmental stage, they die. For example, a juvenile hormone is present in the insect while it is immature. This hormone has been purified by chemists and can be synthesized in the laboratory. If the hormone is applied to an insect in later stages of development, the insect remains "juvenile" and dies. The use of such hormones would be specific to insects, and for this reason they hold promise as a valuable tool for future pest control.

A *pheromone* is a volatile substance secreted in very small amounts by one animal to regulate the behavior of other individuals of the same species. For example, in many species of insects, a virgin female signals her readiness to mate by emitting a small amount of a species-specific chemical sex attractant. The males in the area detect this substance and follow it to its source. Over two dozen insect sex attractants have been isolated and identified in the last decade, and research is now in progress to find out if these natural chemicals can be used to control these insects. One method is to bait traps with small amounts of the pheromones to try to catch the males before they copulate. The problem with this approach is that one must catch almost all the males if the program is to be effective. Another approach is to spray a large area with pheromone so that the smell of virgin females fills the air, leaving the males unable to track down a female. These methods have great potential, for they are species-specific, and only minute amounts of natural, readily degradable chemicals are used; so they cause a minimum of environmental perturbation.

Another method of biological control is the use of sterile mating partners. This technique has been used successfully to eradicate the screwworm (the parasitic larva of the screwworm fly) from the southwestern U.S.A. These larvae are a serious cattle pest, and were causing as much as $40 million damage per year. The females of this fly mate only once during their lifetime, and if they mate with a sterile male, they do not produce fertile eggs. The U.S.D.A. initiated a massive program to rear the flies in the laboratory, irradiating them to render the males sterile, and releasing the sterile males into the natural breeding grounds of the fly. Within a few years the screwworm problem was brought under control in the target areas. Approximately 150 million sterile males are released each week along an 1,800-mile front from the Gulf of Mexico to the Pacific Ocean, at an annual cost of $5 million, which is far less than the economic damage caused by the screwworm. A pilot program is underway to use the sterile-male technique to control the tsetse fly in Africa, which is a serious pest to cattle and humans. Chemical control of the tsetse fly has been reasonably successful in the past, but the fly populations are becoming resistant to insecticides.

In addition to methods for controlling the biology of the pest itself, methods are being developed to control the pest population by the use of its natural enemies. The density of an insect population fluctuates around an equilibrium size (see Figure 8.4). The population rises when there is good weather, ample food, and few natural enemies; it falls when these situations are reversed. This is generally true in both natural and agricultural systems. Insects only become pests when their populations become so large that economic injury to the crop is apparent. We saw earlier that this population increase often occurs in agricultural systems because the crops provide an abundant food supply for the insects. The pest population must now be lowered, by insecticides, for example. Insecticides kill off most of the insects, but the population soon recovers, especially if many pesticide-resistant individuals are already present in the population. Soon the economic injury level will be reached again. However, if the natural balance which keeps the population fluctuating around a certain size is altered, a new equilibrium with a lower population density will be maintained. This can often be achieved by introducing natural enemies that were previously absent from the system (see Figure 8.5). Since the natural enemies have the same diversity as the pests upon which they prey, it is unlikely that resistant pest strains will develop rapidly. Therefore biological control by the introduction of natural enemies is specific and long-lasting.

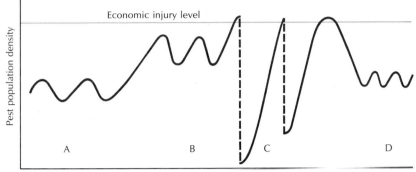

FIGURE 8.4.
Fluctuations in a pest population and its control. A. Before agriculture, the population fluctuates around an equilibrium level. B. After agriculture begins, the additional food for the pest that is provided by the crop allows the pest to establish a higher equilibrium level. Occasionally, the pest population rises above the economic injury level, causing damage to the crop. C. When pesticides are introduced, they kill the pests but also many of their natural enemies; the population of the pest thus rises again until the pesticide is reapplied. Occasionally, pesticide-resistant pests appear. D. When integrated biological and chemical pest control is introduced, a new equilibrium, well below economic injury, is established. (Adapted from R. Smith and R. van den Bosch in Pest Control, *edited by W. Kilgore and R. Doutt, Academic Press, 1967.)*

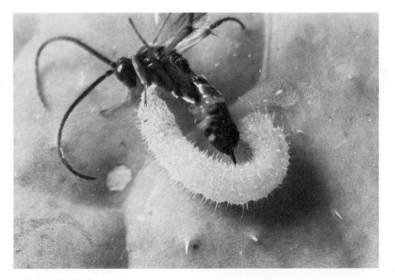

FIGURE 8.5.
An insect parasite attacking a corn earworm. (Photo courtesy of U.S.D.A.)

Table 8.5. Decrease in damage by sugar-cane borer in Barbados after a parasite was introduced in July 1966.[a]

Percent of cane infected	Year
15.0	1966
12.7	1967
9.7	1968
8.0	1969
5.9	1970
4.8	1971

[a]From F. J. Simmonds, "Biological Control of the Sugar-Cane Borer in Barbados," *Entomophaga*, 17 (1972), 251–264.

After the prickly-pear cactus was introduced to Australia in 1890, it grew unchecked because it had no natural enemies. By 1920, this cactus had become a pest, rendering more than 60 million acres of arable land unusable. A natural enemy, an insect, was introduced from Argentina in 1925, and ten years later the cactus had virtually disappeared. In Barbados, the sugar-cane borer worm had caused considerable losses of this crop, a backbone of that island's economy. Introduction from India of an insect parasite of this pest has reduced the previous losses, for a net annual savings of $2 million (see Table 8.5). These are but two of over 100 examples of insect and weed pest control by biological agents. Given the specificity of these methods, it is unfortunate that world expenditures for biological control research are less than 1 percent of those on pesticides.

CHAPTER 9

Plant Breeding and the Green Revolution

There are few more striking examples of how science serves human beings than the way that the principles of heredity are used to provide more food for the human population. To obtain high yields from their crops, farmers can use all the technological inputs available to them. However, irrigation, fertilizers, and pesticides will improve the yield of a given crop strain only to the point at which the plants are making maximum use of the inputs. When the yield plateau is reached for a given strain, little further improvement in yield is possible, because the strain has reached its inherent maximum yield. The major achievement of plant breeding has been to create new strains which have pushed upward the limits of yield.

HEREDITY

The Nature of Variation

There is a great deal of variation among the individuals of a species. Sometimes, this variation is all-or-none: some people have hemophilia (an inherited disease in which blood cannot clot), and others do not; some wheat plants can resist rust fungus, but others cannot. Usually, however, variation is not abrupt, but is continuous in nature. Many plant populations, like human populations, show continuous variation in height. Many plants cluster around an "average" height, but there are also some taller and shorter ones.

It is important for plant breeders to know both the average and the variability in distribution of an agriculturally important trait in a plant population. These two variables can be found experimentally by making measurements on a large population. For example, by measuring the heights of many corn plants, and plotting them on a graph that shows how often each height occurs in the population, one obtains a bell-shaped curve. A hypothetical result for three different strains of corn is shown in Figure 9.1. The frequency distributions of the plant heights immediately reveal two facts: the plants of strain B are, on the average, taller than those of either strain A or strain C; and in strains A and B there is much greater variability (the curves are broader at the base) in the heights of the corn plants than in strain C.

The causes of the variability in height in the corn plant could be that the innate potential of the individuals varies (heredity), or that each plant receives different amounts of nutrients, sunlight, and other environmental variables. Discovering which possibility is correct is a difficult but important task. If heredity is responsible for height, a taller strain of corn could be bred by, for example, selecting tall plants for reproduction. If environment

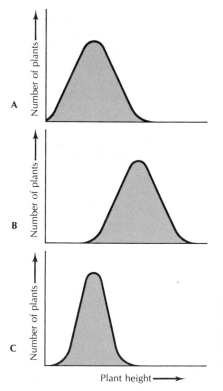

FIGURE 9.1.
Frequency distributions for height of three strains of corn grown under identical conditions. Strains A and C have an identical "average" height, but strain A has a greater variability. Strains A and B have different "average" heights, and similar variability.

is responsible for height, taller plants could be obtained by technological inputs. Unfortunately, the answer lies somewhere between these two possibilities. By growing corn plants in carefully controlled environments, agronomists have found that both heredity and environment determine height. A similar situation exists for many other agriculturally important characteristics, with the relative contributions of heredity and environment being different for different traits (see Table 9.1). Technically speaking, the numerous characteristics by which we recognize an organism constitute its *phenotype*. We recognize a corn plant by the shape and positioning of its leaves, by its size, by the presence of a tassel and an ear, and by many other features. These characteristics constitute the phenotype of the corn plant. Some characteristics of the phenotype are inherited, that is, transmitted from the parent to its offspring; others are environmentally determined; others have both hereditary and environmental causes.

The hereditary elements which help determine the phenotype are called the *genes*. However, plants do not inherit "tallness," but rather the ability to grow tall. They inherit a gene for this ability, and when this gene is fully expressed, the plant will be tall. Thus, genes interacting with the environment determine the phenotype of a plant. In corn, for example, a plant may inherit from its parents the genes for tallness, but, because of inadequate nutrition, drought, or disease, the plant may be short. This fact, that genes represent potential and not actual characteristics (phenotype), is crucial to agriculture. Plant breeders can develop new strains of crops which move the yield plateau ever upward, but the plateau will not be reached if even one of the many requirements for healthy plant growth is not met.

Table 9.1. Heredity and environment.[a]

Characteristic	Per cent determined by	
	Heredity	Environment
Conception rate in cattle	5	95
Ear length in corn	17	83
Egg production in poultry	20	80
Yield in corn	25	75
Oil content in corn	65	35
Egg weight in poultry	60	40
Root length in radishes	65	35
Slaughter weight in cattle	85	15

[a]From J. Brewbaker, *Agricultural Genetics*, © 1964. Reprinted by permission of Prentice-Hall, Inc., Englewood Cliffs, N.J.

Inheritance of Genes

Although its genes may give a corn plant the potential to grow tall, a population of plants placed in the same environment will often show variation in height. One reason for this variation is that genes can change, and when these changes are permanent and passed on to the next generation, they are termed mutations. Mutations occur very rarely, but after a long period of time they can account for quite a bit of variability in a population. For example, a gene which determines the height of a corn plant may have mutated in one plant to a form which confers on that plant the potential to grow taller than normal. In another plant, a mutation could exist for shortness. In this way, the continuous variation in height can be thought of as the sum of many changes which occurred because of gene mutations.

The second, and most important, factor that creates genetic variation in a population is that most animals and plants possess two copies of every gene. Genes are located in filamentous structures in the cell nucleus called *chromosomes.* The chromosomes are discrete structures which become visible under the light microscope when a cell undergoes the process of cell division. Most cells probably have many thousands of genes, although there are not nearly as many chromosomes. Thus, hundreds or even thousands of genes can be located on a single chromosome. Most higher organisms have two copies of every chromosome in every cell, except for the sex cells. In humans each cell has 23 pairs of chromosomes, for a total of 46. Corn has 10 pairs of chromosomes, and Happlopappus, a small desert plant, has only two pairs. Cells which have two copies of every chromosome therefore also have two copies of every gene on those chromosomes. When these two copies are identical, the organism is said to be *homozygous* for that gene. If one of the two copies has mutated, they will be different, and this condition is termed *heterozygous.*

The chromosomes play a vital role in passing on genes, and therefore phenotypic characteristics, from a mother cell to the daughter cells, when an organism is growing by cell division, and from the parents to the offspring during reproduction.

The process of passing on genes may be followed in Figure 9.2, which is for an organism with only two pairs of chromosomes. Let us first consider the simpler case of cell division, or *mitosis,* which normally occurs in meristems (Chapter 3). How does a mother cell insure that the two daughter cells will have two copies of every gene? If all the genes were structurally separate from one another, it could be quite difficult to sort out two sets of several thousand genes and make sure that one set ends up in each daugh-

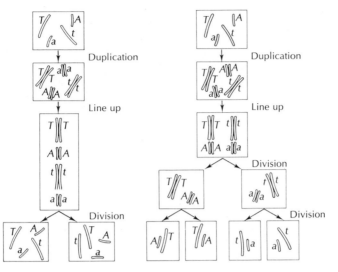

FIGURE 9.2.
Mitosis (left) and meiosis (right) in an organism that has two chromosome pairs and is heterozygous for two genes.

ter cell. Because the genes are located on the chromosomes, the cell only has to have a mechanism to sort out and separate two sets of chromosomes.

Before mitosis begins, the cell in Figure 9.2 contains in its nucleus two pairs of chromosomes, for a total of four. Let us consider this organism to be heterozygous for two pairs of genes, *Tt* (located on the long chromosome) and *Aa* (located on the short chromosome). The first step in mitosis is a duplication of each chromosome. This doubling actually occurs before the chromosomes are visible as microscopically discrete structures. Thus when the chromosomes do become visible, they appear as double strands, already containing two copies of each of their genes. At that point the cell contains four copies of each gene. During the subsequent stages of mitosis, these doubled strands line up at the center of the cell and split longitudinally, a single strand of each pair going to one end of the cell, and its sister strand to the other end of the cell. Since the two strands are identical copies of the same, original genes, this means that the two new cells which form will contain the identical genetic complement of the cell from which they came. Each daughter cell will have two copies of every gene. If the two copies were different, then those differences would be passed on from the mother cell to the daughter cells.

During the formation of eggs and sperm, a different type of cell division occurs. An organism passes on to its sex cells only one copy of every gene. When two sex cells fuse during fertilization to start a new organism, the cells of this new organism will again contain two copies of every gene. A plant homozygous for a given gene will produce sex cells all of which have identical forms of that gene; that is, in terms of that gene, it produces only one type of reproductive cell. However, a plant heterozygous for a gene, with, for example, one normal and one mutant copy, will produce two types of reproductive cells: half the sex cells will carry the normal gene, half will carry the mutant gene.

This process, called reduction division—the total number of chromosomes is "reduced" to half—or *meiosis,* is carried out by separation of chromosomes. It may be followed for our *TtAa* plant on the righthand side of Figure 9.2. The first phase of meiosis is identical to that of mitosis: the chromosomes duplicate themselves, and each one becomes a double strand. These double-stranded chromosomes now line up in the center of the cell in such a way that two homologous or look-alike chromosomes line up beside each other. In the next step, these two look-alike chromosomes separate and move to opposite poles of the cell, each chromosome in its double-stranded form. The resulting two daughter cells have only half as many chromosomes as the mother cell. This separation of chromosomes is the fundamental difference between mitosis and meiosis, for in mitosis the two strands of each chromosome separate and move to opposite poles of the cell. In meiosis, when these double-stranded chromosomes migrate to the ends of the cell, they do not split, as in mitosis, but one doubled chromosome of each pair goes to each end of the cell. This process is followed by mitosis without an intervening duplication of the chromosomes. Thus four sex cells are formed, each with a single copy of each chromosome and gene. In this way a parent passes only one of its two copies of each gene to its offspring, and the offspring inherits one copy of each gene from its maternal parent and one from its paternal parent. This is obviously one way in which an organism can become heterozygous for a given gene.

As an example, suppose that height variation in corn plants is caused by a single gene with two different forms: T confers tallness and t confers shortness. These two forms of the gene can occur in three different combinations in the plant. Plants may be homozygous for T (TT or tall phenotype), homozygous for t (tt or short phenotype), or heterozygous (Tt or average phenotype). Meiosis in the tall plants leads to sex cells that have only the T gene, in the short plants to cells that have only the t gene. However, plants of average height produce two kinds of sex cells, half with *T* genes, half with *t* genes. When these average plants breed among themselves, the results are as shown in Figure 9.3: ¼ of the offspring will be tall, ¼ will be short, and ½ will be of average height. Thus plants of a given pheontype do not necessarily beget plants of the same phenotype.

As the number of independent gene pairs in a heterozygous organism increases, the possible number of different reproductive cells increases. In the example in the preceding paragraph, plants with one heterozygous gene pair could pass on either of two types of sex cells in a given mating. In the hypothetical *TtAa* plant of Figure 9.2, there are four types of sex cells possible. During meiosis, the double strands line up with homologous chromosomes side by side, and it is entirely random which of the homologous pair goes to which end of the cell. Although the drawing shows that the *TT* and *AA* chromosomes went to one end and *tt* and *aa* to the other, it is equally probable that the *TT* and *aa* chromosomes could go to one end, and *tt* and *AA* to the other. Thus *TtAa* plants could produce the following types of sex cells: *TA, ta, Ta,* or *tA.* If there are three gene pairs involved, there are eight possible combinations; if there are four gene pairs involved, the or-

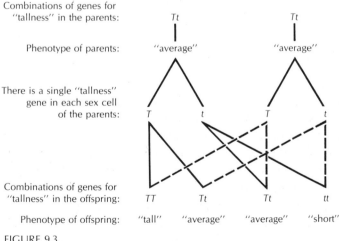

FIGURE 9.3.
Random inheritance of genes. Each parent has two copies of the gene for tallness. The gene can exist in one of two forms: T or t. Only one form of the gene from each parent appears in an individual sex cell and in each offspring. It is random which form of the gene from one parent combines with that of the other.

ganism can produce 16 different types of sex cells; and so on. Since many genes in an organism are heterozygous, the parents can make many genetically different reproductive cells, and the number of different offspring from any two parents can obviously be quite large. For example, the *TtAa* plants mentioned above, could, if bred among themselves, produce offspring that have nine different gene combinations for these two particular gene pairs. If one considers four different gene pairs, all heterozygous, the possible combinations number 81. The fact that plants are normally heterozygous for many genes creates numerous possibilities for variation in the offspring because of random recombination of genes during fertilization. A third factor which leads to variation in a population of organisms is that many genes affect a single phenotypic characteristic. For example, among the more important genetic characteristics which determine yield are disease resistance, ability to take up soil nutrients and respond to fertilizer, photosynthetic efficiency, and seed size. Each of these is determined by many genes. For example, responsiveness to nitrogen fertilizers involves genes which regulate the uptake of nitrate by the roots, the conversion of nitrate to ammonium in the plant body, the translocation of amino acids to the developing seeds and the biosynthesis of seed proteins. To sort out the combinations of genes involved in agriculturally important characteristics is the challenge facing the plant breeder.

METHODS OF PLANT BREEDING

Pure-Line Selection

Knowledge of the laws of heredity permits a more precise explanation of the selection methods used by the early farmers who domesticated crops (Chapter 6). Most of the wild relatives of modern crop plants show considerable variability for many traits. Domestication involved the selection from the extremes of the distribution curve (Figure 9.1) for the phenotype desired. In the domestication of wheat, the early farmers selected for plants with tough spikes from a population in which toughness of spike was a variable characteristic. After many generations of selecting plants and breeding the selected plants to each other (inbreeding), the frequency-distribution curve for spike roughness looked quite different from the original one for wild plants. First, the average was shifted to tougher spikes, and, second, the amount of variability was reduced, so that the distribution curve became narrower.

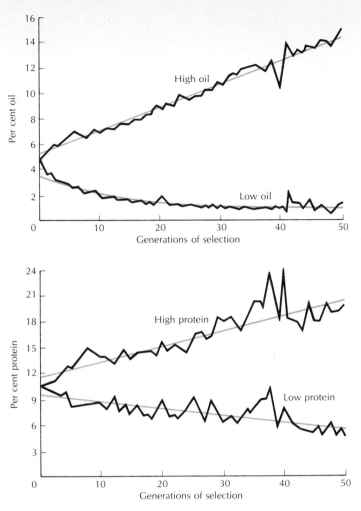

FIGURE 9.4.
Selection for oil content and protein content in corn. The solid lines indicate actual data, the grey lines, trends. Thus in a comparatively short time, people can use genetic variability to select strains of a desired phenotype. (U.S.D.A.)

In genetic terms, a selected and inbred population is more homozygous than its wild relatives. Thinking back to the corn-height phenotypes discussed above, we can see that the early farmers selected for reproduction only *TT* plants, those which had the desired phenotype and which would always pass on the gene for that phenotype. Thus, after a long time, a crop which in the wild had been heterozygous and had exhibited great variability became a homozygous pure line which would always "breed true" to its phenotype. An example of a modern experiment to select a pure line is shown in Figure 9.4, where corn was selected and bred for oil and protein content in the grain. Once again, note that defined phenotypes, at the extremes of the frequency-distribution curve, are selected.

There are two problems with pure-line selection as a method for crop improvement. One problem is that, as the plants become homozygous for the desired genes, they may also become homozygous for some harmful genes which were previously "masked" by being present in a heterozygous plant. Thus selection for tough spikes may also mean an unknowing selection for plants susceptible to rust because the genes for both phenotypes were present in the same plant. The other, related problem with pure-line selection is that it reduces variability in other possibly beneficial characteristics. For example, there may have been genes for disease resistance in the wild wheat population, but human selection for tough spikes eliminated this beneficial characteristic.

Hybridization

In 1908, the American breeder G. H. Shull reported the results of crossing corn plants from two different pure lines. The cross between these two homozygous lines produced a heterozygous offspring, because the lines were homozygous for different sets of genes. The result was astonishing. The two inbred lines had each produced about 20 bushels of corn per acre in the last crop. Their outbred offspring quadrupled this yield, to 80 bushels per acre! This unanticipated strength in the heterozygous outcross was called "hybrid vigor" and such hybrids have played a great role in increasing yield (see Table 9.2). By 1919, the first commercial hybrid corn was available in the U.S., and two decades later nearly all the corn was hybrid, as it is to this day. Similar experiments led to the development of hybrid sorghum (1957), millet (1959), barley (1969), and cotton (1970), although these four are not yet commercial successes.

Table 9.2. Hybrid corn and yields.[a]

Corn strain	Yield in bushels per acre
"Original"	80
Inbred, after 30 generations	20
Hybrid of inbreds	75
Offspring of hybrid	40

[a]From J. Brewbaker, *Agricultural Genetics*, © 1964. Reprinted by permission of Prentice-Hall, Inc., Englewood Cliffs, N.J.

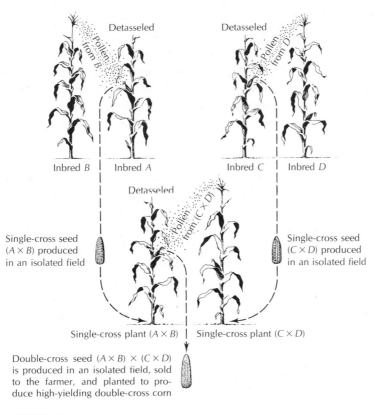

Single-cross seed
($A \times B$) produced
in an isolated field

Single-cross seed
($C \times D$) produced
in an isolated field

Single-cross plant ($A \times B$) | Single-cross plant ($C \times D$)

Double-cross seed ($A \times B$) $\times$ ($C \times D$)
is produced in an isolated field, sold
to the farmer, and planted to produce high-yielding double-cross corn

FIGURE 9.5.
Method of producing hybrid corn and representative ears of the crop produced from hybrid seed. Most of the corn now grown in the U.S. is produced by this "double-cross" method.

The first step in hybrid production is to generate homozygous, inbred lines. This is normally done by means of self-pollinating plants, where pollen from male flowers fertilizes female flowers on the same plant. When this is repeated for many generations, and as the number of homozygous gene pairs thus increases, a decline in yield sets in, usually because deleterious genes become homozygous during the selection process. Once the pure lines are generated, they are outcrossed, and the original high yield is restored. If the object of this procedure is to get the original yield, why not use the "original" plants? This would certainly work, but we would soon run out of "original" plants, and since they are heterozygous for many gene pairs, reproducing them would yield extremely variable seeds. What hybridization does is to make high yield dependable. The inbred lines breed true and can be kept forever, theoretically, in this genetic state.

A problem with hybridization is that the farmer must buy new hybrid seed crop every year, and cannot use part of his own crop as seed corn for the following spring. The plants which grow from the hybrid seeds cross-pollinate and produce a bumper crop as a result of hybrid vigor. However, seeds of the crop are highly heterozygous, and when they are planted there is much variability among the plants and in their ability to produce seeds. Thus, hybrid vigor rapidly disappears in successive generations. Development of the inbred strains and production of hybrid seed require knowledge, time, and money, and these services are provided by seed companies which sell their seeds to the farmer. The widespread use of hybrid corn seed has kept the price of seed down, and the extra income generated by the greater corn yield is much greater than the price of the seed. For other hybrids which are not yet widely planted, the hybrid seed is still quite expensive, and this expense prevents its adoption by the smaller farmers.

Backcrossing

Backcrossing makes it possible to transfer specific genes from one plant strain to another. In this way, desirable characteristics of one strain can be combined with those of another strain. This trick circumvents the problem of trying to select simultaneously for many traits in the same strain.

Tall wheat plants, when they are heavily fertilized with nitrogen, fall over at maturity because the slender stalk is unable to bear the heavy load of grain. As a result, much of the harvest can be lost, especially if the wheat is harvested by combine. For this reason, plant breeders have tried to breed shorter strains of cereals. Suppose one wants to introduce, by backcrossing, a gene for "shortness" into a normal, high-yielding, tall wheat strain (see Figure 9.6). First, one finds a suitable wheat strain which is short. It may not have any other desirable characteristics, such as high yield, but that does not really matter. The short strain is crossed with the normal tall wheat, and from the offspring one selects those plants which are most like the original high-yielding strain, but which also have the gene for shortness. These plants are then crossed again with the short strain and again one selects plants which resemble the original high-yielding strain, but are also short.

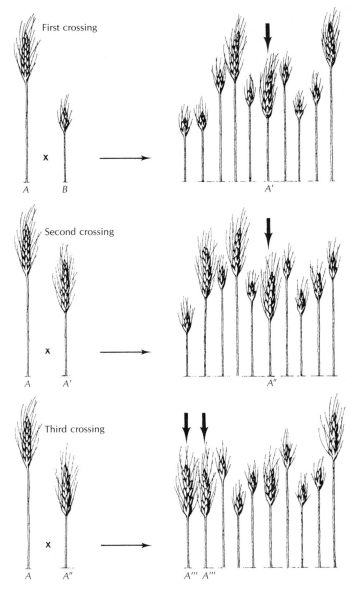

FIGURE 9.6.
Hypothetical scheme for backcrossing. The objective is to introduce the gene for shortness from strain B into the high-yielding wheat strain, A. From the first cross of A × B, plants (A') are selected which resemble A but are shorter. These are crossed to the initial strain, A. Once again, plants (A'') are selected which resemble A but are shorter. These in turn are crossed back to strain A. After repeated crossing and selections, the gene for shortness of strain B becomes part of strain A.

This backcrossing selection procedure is repeated five to ten times, until a new strain of wheat emerges, one that has all the desirable characteristics of the original strain and also has the gene for shortness.

Backcrossing has been valuable for introducing such characteristics as height and disease resistance into crop strains. These phenotypes are best searched for where plant variation is greatest, in the wild populations. Plant breeders continuously search the world for wild relatives of crop plants with desirable characteristics. These wild relatives are especially important in breeding for disease resistance, because new disease strains are constantly arising.

Introduction of Mutations

Mutations create genetic variability, but the natural rate of permanent gene changes is quite slow. Indeed, it has probably taken millions of years to achieve the variability observed in natural populations of crop plants. Within the last half-century, geneticists have found ways to speed up this mutation process greatly. Both radiation (such as X-rays) and certain chemicals can, by modifying gene chemistry, induce mutations. When large numbers of seeds are so treated, mutations of genes are induced at random. Most of these gene changes are harmful, but a tiny number may be beneficial. Thousands of seeds must be treated and planted and screened to detect, possibly, one good mutation which can then be bred into the crop plant by backcrossing.

Induced mutations have had a great impact on agriculture. For example, Indian scientists were able to breed a strain of castor bean that matures in 120 days instead of the usual 270; this allows an extra crop per year on the same land. Italians created a strong, short-stemmed durum wheat (the kind used to make pasta) which will not fall over in the field when given large amounts of fertilizer. Japanese breeders are inducing mutations in rice which, they hope, will cause protein to be distributed throughout the grain, not just in the germ and outer layers, which are removed when rice is polished. Success in this project will mean a great improvement in the protein diets of millions of people.

Polyploid Breeding

Organisms with more than two copies of every gene are termed *polyploids*. This condition can arise spontaneously in nature or can be artificially induced by specific chemicals. In nature, polyploids usually arise from sex cells that have extra sets of chromosomes. For example, chromosomes may fail to migrate to the ends of the cell, so that during meiosis one end of the cell receives all the chromosomes, and the other end none; this results in the formation of a sex cell which has two chromosome sets. When this cell combines with a sex cell that has a single set of chromosomes during fertilization, the resulting organism will have three sets of chromosomes.

Polyploids have played a major role in the evolution of modern crop plants. Plant strains which early farmers selected for their vigorous growth or high yield often turned out to be polyploids. For some plants, increases in the number of chromosome sets are correlated with increases in the sizes of leaves, stems, fruits, and flowers. This is especially true for ornamentals, such as petunias, where there are series of both wild and cultivated varieties which show both larger flowers and additional chromosome sets.

In addition to the duplication of chromosome sets in a single species, polyploids can arise from the combination of chromosomes from two different species. For example, the modern plum tree is diploid, with two sets of 24 chromosomes; eight of these chromosomes represent the complement of the cherry plum, and the other 16 represent the complement of the blackthorn. The additional chromosomes in the modern plum lead to larger fruit and a higher yield. In a similar manner, modern tobacco, a diploid with two sets of 24 chromosomes, is believed to have arisen from two lower-yielding species with twelve chromosomes each. Many modern wheat strains are polyploid, and the evolution of modern wheats from their wild relatives in terms of chromosomes parallels that of agricultural selection (see Figure 6.3). Early diploid wheat, einkorn, has fourteen chromosomes (two sets of seven), which are designated AA. This species is believed to have hybridized with a wild grass species to produce emmer wheat. The latter, now common as durum or pasta wheat, has the AA chromosome sets and the BB sets of the wild grass. This tetraploid, $AABB$, now mated with yet another wild grass species, which had the chromosome complement designated DD, to yield $AABBDD$, our modern hexaploid wheat, which has 42 chromosomes. The two wild grasses that contributed the B and D chromosomes to this evolutionary scheme have been identified as goat-grasses endemic to Turkey and the region of the Fertile Crescent. Thus it is not surprising to find agricultural beginnings in this area.

Some polyploids are unable to reproduce sexually and do not produce seeds. Generally, these plants have an odd number of chromosome sets. Formation of sex cells involves a splitting of the diploid cell such that each sex cell receives one-half of the diploid complement, or one copy of each gene. This packaging machinery breaks down in a triploid, for example, since a sex cell can receive only a full chromosome complement, not half of one. Thus the inability to make viable sex cells renders such plants sterile. This can be an advantage, as in the production of seedless fruits, such as watermelons. But it is a disadvantage in that the plants must be propagated asexually and bred by grafting. Many apple, pear, and citrus varieties are triploid, and thus must be propagated asexually.

An important extension of polyploid breeding has been the development of the wheat-rye hybrid called triticale. This resulted from an attempt to combine the high yield and high seed-protein content of wheat with the adaptability to adverse environmental conditions (such as cold and drought) and high seed-lysine content of rye. The initial cross was made in 1889, but the plants were sterile, because the hybrid had one copy of the wheat chromosomes (ABD) and one copy of the rye (F). Thus, when the resulting plant ($ABDF$) attempted to form sex cells, there was no way for the gametes to receive both one copy of every gene and half the copies of the parent plant. Recently, methods were developed to treat triticale seedlings chemically so that they would double their chromosomes. The resulting plants ($AABBDDFF$) are fully fertile, and their offspring are likewise fertile. Currently, a worldwide research program sponsored by the Canadian International Research Center is underway to attempt to develop triticale into a major grain crop.

AIMS OF CROP IMPROVEMENT

The aim of crop improvement is to create new strains which yield more food of better nutritional value than their predecessors. In previous chapters, we described the physiological bases for food production by plants, as well as the environmental requirements for the optimal functioning of the plants. Now, with the tools of the plant breeder at hand, we can decide what desirable attributes crop plants should have. For which phenotypes are we breeding?

1. High primary productivity   A high primary productivity is almost invariably related to a high crop yield. High productivity can be achieved by ensuring that all the light which falls on the field is intercepted by the leaves, and that photosynthesis itself is as efficient as possible. Greater efficiency in photosynthesis could perhaps be achieved by selecting against photorespiration (Chapter 4).

2. High crop yield   In a world of food shortages, people need crop plants that produce more food per cultivated area. Plants must be selected which turn a high proportion of their total primary productivity into the plant parts which people eat (whether seeds, roots, or stems). The plants must also be strong enough to bear the crop.

3. High nutritional quality   Higher crop yield is more beneficial to people if the nutritional qualities of the crops can be maintained or improved. The amounts of certain essential amino acids and the total protein in cereal grains should be increased to improve their nutritional quality. The same should be done with "root crops," such as potatoes, sweet potatoes, and cassava.

4. Efficient absorption of soil minerals   Plants with a genetic capacity for high yields use large amounts of plant nutrients to produce those yields. Thus, they can respond to added fertilizers. Plants should be selected which can obtain more nutrients from the soil because the nutrient carriers in the membranes of the root cells have a higher affinity for the nutrients.

5. More extensive and efficient nitrogen fixation   Strains of nitrogen-fixing bacteria which are more efficient at providing the plant with fixed nitrogen are being developed. Cereal grains which have nitrogen-fixing microorganisms living in the soil around their roots will require less nitrogen fertilizer.

6. More efficient use of water and drought resistance   Crop plants which use water more efficiently (have a smaller transpiration ratio) and which are resistant to drought are now being developed. This is important because many areas of the world have insufficient rainfall to allow use of the strains now in existence.

7. Resistance to pests   If all crop plants were resistant to pests, food production would rise dramatically. Breeding for pest resistance is an on-going concern, because new strains of pests, especially fungi, always arise and attack the plants which were resistant to the old strains.

8. Insensitivity to photoperiod   Many crop plants flower and set seed in response to daylength (Chapter 3). This phenomenon limits the plants to a certain climatic zone and limits harvest to once a year. Selection of crop strains which are insensitive to photoperiod or are adapted to a variety of photoperiods would allow multiple cropping during a growing season.

9. Plant architecture and adaptability to mechanized farming
The number and positioning of the leaves, the branching pattern of the

stem, the height of the plant, and the positioning of the organs to be harvested are all important to crop production. They often determine how well plants will intercept light, how closely they can be planted, and how easily the crop can be harvested mechanically.

Clearly, crop improvement means an attack on all these fronts. We have described already some of the progress in and prospects for improving productivity, nitrogen fixation, and disease resistance. In the last decade or so, dramatic advances have been made, and are continuing in the improvement of quality and yields.

IMPROVING QUALITY: HIGH-LYSINE CORN AND SORGHUM

Corn is the staple of people in 14 countries of Latin America and sub-Saharan Africa. In addition, it is an important feed grain for cattle and hogs in many developed countries. Corn protein does not supply adequate amounts of all the amino acids essential for the human diet: it is especially deficient in lysine and, to a lesser extent, tryptophan. For this reason, those people who receive their dietary protein from corn often suffer from protein malnutrition.

In 1963, during screening of many corn varieties for protein quality, U.S. scientists found that grains carrying a gene called "opaque-2" were higher in lysine and tryptophan than is normal corn. Their relative quantities of other amino acids were about normal; so the new strain was named "high-lysine corn." Realizing immediately the possible nutritive value of their discovery, the scientists fed diets of normal or opaque-2 corn (supplemented with vitamins and minerals) to baby rats. The rats on the opaque-2 diet gained nearly four times as much weight as those on normal corn! Similar tests were run on hogs, with the same result. Soon opaque-2 corn meal was being used in Colombia to cure children of kwashiorkor. Currently this corn meal is being marketed in that country as the first food an infant should eat after being weaned from mother's milk. Considerable progress is reported in its use in preventing protein malnutrition.

The opaque-2 gene poses a challenge for the plant breeder. The originally screened strains were low-yielding and had a sweet taste, soft texture, and color that were unappealing to consumers. Breeders were asked to breed the nutritious high-lysine gene into commercial varieties which have high yields and consumer acceptance. Considerable progress has been made, and the conversion of many corn strains to opaque-2 strains is underway.

Sorghum is the world's fourth most important cereal crop. It can withstand drought better than many other crops (for example, corn), and so can be grown on soils unsuitable for cultivation of other crops. Although in the U.S. it is primarily used as an animal feed, in Africa and east Asia millions of people use sorghum seeds as a dietary staple. However, sorghum protein, like that of corn, is deficient in lysine. In 1973, Drs. R. Singh and J. Axtell of Purdue University announced the result of a biochemical screening program similar to that undertaken for corn a decade earlier: two of the 9,000 strains of sorghum examined had nutritionally adequate amounts of lysine in the grain protein (see Table 9.3). Tests using young rats showed that the high-lysine sorghum promoted three times the weight gain produced by normal sorghum. Field tests are underway in the U.S. and India which may bring these high-lysine sorghum strains to the consumer.

In 1969, the Swedish scientist L. Munck reported a high-lysine, high-protein barley strain called Hiproly. Two additional strains have been found in an experiment in which mutations were induced with chemicals. A breeding program is currently underway to introduce these high-lysine genes into commercial varieties of barley.

At the Nebraska agricultural experiment station, plant geneticists reported in 1974 that three strains of wheat possess higher protein and lysine contents than most other wheats. Most wheat varieties average about 12 percent protein in the grain, but the new varieties range up to 20 percent in field tests. Whereas many normal wheats average about 2.9 grams of lysine per 100 grams of grain protein, the new varieties average about 3.4 grams. Clearly, breeding these genes for high protein and lysine into the world's wheat crop would be a major nutritional advance for mankind.

Table 9.3. High-lysine corn and sorghum. Amino acid contents as grams per 100 grams of protein.

	Lysine	Tryptophan
Normal corn[a]	2.7	0.7
Opaque-2 corn[a]	4.0	1.3
Normal sorghum[b]	2.0	0.9
High-lysine sorghum[b]	3.3	1.7

[a]Data from E. Mertz, *Proceedings of the Third International Conference on Food-Science Technology* (1971), p. 306.

[b]Data from R. Singh and J. Axtell, "High-Lysine Mutant Gene that Improves Quality and Biological Value of Grain Sorghum," *Crop Science* 13 (1973), 535–539.

IMPROVING YIELDS: THE GREEN REVOLUTION

The Nobel Peace Prize was awarded in 1970 to an American, Norman Borlaug, for his role in the breeding of new, high-yielding strains of wheat. Until that time, few people had ever heard of Borlaug or the new wheat strains. The award, and the inevitable publicity surrounding it, served to tell the world that a new agricultural revolution had begun in the poor countries. This breakthrough in food production has been termed the green revolution. It represents the culmination so far of our attempts to use the principles of breeding and agricultural science to improve crops.

The New Wheats

From the time of plant domestication, people selected for and bred tall wheat strains. These may have been easier for the primitive farmers to harvest, or, as some psychologists suggest, they may have provided a symbol of fertility. At any rate, such tall-stalked plants were not suited for high yields. When they produced a great number of seeds, the slender stalks would fall over (lodge), and the seeds then couldn't be harvested. One object of breeding the new wheats, then, was to breed high-yielding strains with short, tough stalks that wouldn't lodge.

The origin and development of the new wheats is represented in Figure 9.7. In Japan, semidwarf wheat strains had been developed by selection. To improve the yields of these strains, the Japanese decided to cross them with higher-yielding American varieties. In 1917, a series of crosses was made with the Japanese Daruma and American Fultz strains. The offspring of these crosses, selected for both Daruma dwarfness and high yield, were again crossed with the American strains in a type of backcross. By 1935, one of the products of these crosses, Norin 10, was made available to farmers and greatly increased yields were reported. After the Second World War, the agricultural advisor to the American occupation army in Japan saw the success of Norin 10 and brought some seeds back to the U.S. Soon, workers in the U.S. Pacific Northwest were breeding the Japanese semidwarf with their local wheats in order to confer on it genes which could adapt it to their local conditions. A result was Gaines wheat: short, strong, high-yielding, and well-adapted to the heavy rainfall of that region. Again, record wheat yields were reported.

There were two problems with Gaines wheat that made it unsuitable for growing in tropical and semitropical climates. First, it was a winter wheat. This means that it is planted in the fall and harvested in the spring.

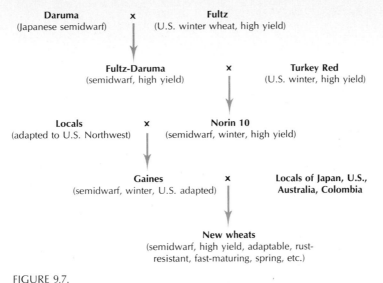

FIGURE 9.7.
Origin of the new wheats. Each "cross" represents many actual crosses to fix the new characteristics into the strains.

Winter wheats need a period of cold during early growth, and if they do not get this cold period, they will not produce grain. This, of course, precluded using Gaines wheat in the countries of Asia, where people needed its extra yields. A second problem was its susceptibility to rust. Large dusting programs were needed to prevent infection, and, even so, during epidemics yields plummeted.

In 1953, some Gaines seeds and others from similar Norin 10 crosses were sent to Dr. Borlaug in Mexico. Working under the auspices of the Rockefeller Foundation, he and his colleagues set up breeding criteria for the wheat strains to make them adaptable to the growing conditions of the poor countries. (These criteria were similar to the ones we set out earlier in this chapter.) By collecting many varieties of wheat seeds from all around the world, they amassed a great "gene bank" from which they could breed into the semidwarfs desirable characteristics, such as adaptability to different climates. These crosses were made and grown at two locations in Mexico. One, Toluca, is on a high (2,500 meters above sea level) plateau near Mexico City; the other, Ciudad Obregon, is in the hotter state of Sonora (see Figure 9.8). Choice of these two sites did two things for the breeding effort: first, they allowed two growing seasons a year, thus speeding up experimentation; and second, they allowed selection of strains adaptable to both cool and hot climates.

By 1963, the Mexico breeding project had produced new, high-yielding, semidwarf strains with important new characteristics. They were spring wheats, meaning that they were planted in spring and harvested in

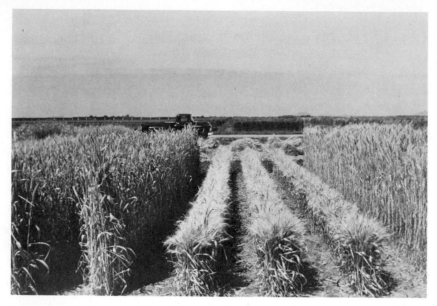

FIGURE 9.8.
*Semidwarf wheat (in the center) growing near Ciudad Obregon, Mexico. Notice
the standard tall wheat on either side. (Photo courtesy of U.S.D.A.)*

summer. Where winters are mild, however, such wheats can also be planted
in fall and harvested in spring, thus potentially allowing two crops a year.
The new strains matured quickly and were insensitive to photoperiod, two
traits also conducive to multiple cropping. They were rust-resistant, and
they were well-adapted to a variety of warm climates. Borlaug sent 100 kilograms of these seeds to the government of India in 1963, and a decade later
one third of India's wheat acreage and half of that of Pakistan was planted
with the new strains.

The New Rices

At about the same time that the Mexican wheats were being developed,
plant breeders were hard at work improving the yields and properties of
the other main staple of the world, rice. Much of this research was done
in India and Japan, but it culminated with the development of new, high-
yielding rice strains at the International Rice Research Institute in the
Philippines.

The story of rice breeding is much like that of wheat. Most Asians ate, and still eat, Indica rice, a strain well-adapted to low soil fertility and monsoon agriculture. This rice has been selected for high disease resistance, and the grains have the dry cooking characteristics preferred by the people of these regions. But the crop matures slowly, so that multiple cropping is impossible, and the plants are tall, so that they will lodge if they produce a high yield of seeds.

In the 1950's, significant steps were taken to improve the Indica strains. In Indonesia, outcrosses to local varieties produced Peta, a higher-yielding, relatively drought-resistant strain. In Taiwan, extensive breeding of Dee-geo-woo-gen, a semidwarf variety, with local Indicas yielded TN-1, a strain which responded well to fertilizer by increasing yields and, since it had a short stalk, did not lodge. Then, in the Philippines, breeders crossed Peta with Dee-geo-woo-gen and got "miracle rice," IR-8. Further crosses between TN-1 and Peta yielded another strain, IR-20, which was released for use in 1969. Because IR-8 has hard grains after cooking, consumer acceptance has been slow. To overcome this problem, breeders crossed IR-8 with Sigadis, a strain whose grains are soft after cooking, and in 1971 the result, a more acceptable IR-24, was released. In 1973, IR-26, a cross between IR-24 and a disease-resistant TN-1 relative, was released for planting. This strain combines the best characteristics of high yield, consumer acceptability, and disease resistance.

The semidwarf rice strains have revolutionized rice production by doubling yields in some regions. Like the new wheats, they are highly responsive to fertilizer, do not lodge, and mature quite quickly. Farmers and consumers have been enthusiastic about the new rice, and they are rapidly replacing the local Indicas. By 1974, the new strains were being grown on 18 percent of the rice fields of India, 15 percent of those of Indonesia, and almost half of those in Pakistan.

The Green Revolution in China

With the improvements in China's communications with other countries since the early 1970's, it has become apparent that the People's Republic of China has been an active participant in the green revolution. The Chinese population is growing at the rate of 1.1 percent per year, but agricultural production is growing at double this rate. Since 1966, China has been self-sufficient in cereal grains, and in 1973 she was second among the world's nations in the amount of rice exported (the U.S. was first). One can appreciate the magnitude of the Chinese achievement better by considering that the amount of arable land in China is a bit less than that in the U.S., yet China feeds roughly four times the number of people in the American population. Most of the arable land in the eastern half of China is now under cultivation. Thus, the current emphasis on agriculture is to increase yields. Plans are to double grain production during the next 20 years.

An important factor in increasing yields has been the breeding of high-yielding varieties of crops. China initiated its own rice-breeding program in 1956, and produced rice strains very similar to those which were developed at the International Rice Research Institute in the Philippines. Dwarf strains were put into production in 1960, and the amount of acreage planted with them has been increasing. The Chinese also purchased samples of the IRRI rices, such as IR-5 and IR-8, and these have now been crossed with local varieties. In addition to rice, the Chinese have developed their own high-yielding wheat varieties and have imported many of the strains developed in Mexico. Finally, they have developed faster-maturing and higher-yielding strains of soybeans than had been previously planted. This last development has aroused much interest in the U.S., where the few soybean strains under cultivation were originally imported from China and have hardly been improved.

A second factor in the Chinese agricultural success has been an increased use of inorganic fertilizers. Traditionally, soil fertility has been maintained by the use of human and animal wastes or of crop residues which are plowed into the soil. Intensive agricultural practices have demanded that the faster-acting inorganic fertilizers be used. Until the early 1970's, this fertilizer had to be imported; in 1973, for example, China imported 1.8 million tons of nitrogen fertilizer. Recently, however, she has begun a drive to become self-sufficient in this important input. By 1978, a complex of plants are projected to be synthesizing 2.7 million tons of nitrogen fertilizer annually, an amount which should ensure domestic needs and possibly allow for exports. The energy required to synthesize this fertilizer will come from domestic supplies of coal, oil, and natural gas.

China has long been known for the high proportion of its arable land that is irrigated (33 percent, compared to 10 percent in the U.S.) This fact reflects the extreme importance of controlled water supplies for high-intensity agriculture. Recent developments in this endeavor have centered on tube wells (over 300,000 are now in existence), and massive tapping of the watershed by damming and diversion. For example, 90,000 acres of former desert in Sinkiang province are now arable because of the diversion of the Tarim River. These schemes require both labor and mechanization, and neither has been in short supply in China. Over 80 percent of the population is involved in food production, and the political system permits massive mobilizations for such projects. The government runs a large number of plants for farm-machinery manufacture, but many communes are setting up their own repair and manufacturing plants.

CHAPTER 10

The Impact of the Green Revolution

The term "Green Revolution" was coined in the late 1960's to describe the impact of the new high-yielding wheat and rice strains, and of their associated agricultural technologies, on the food-production capacities of several developing countries. Since that time the Green Revolution has been both praised and damned. In the late 1960's, as use of the new strains spread rapidly in Asia, optimism was the rule, and claims were made that many underdeveloped countries would soon be self-sufficient in, and even exporters of, cereal grains. But in the early 1970's, poor weather and global economic constraints slowed the progress of the revolution considerably. The possibility that population growth would soon outstrip the world's capacity to produce food was once again apparent. Pessimists proclaimed that the green revolution had been oversold by the developed nations and overbrought by the developing nations, and that mass starvation was inevitable. As in many scientific controversies, the truth lies somewhere between the extremes of optimism and despair. In this chapter, we examine the progress, impact, and limitations of the green revolution.

CYCLES OF AGRICULTURAL TECHNOLOGY

Agricultural economists have shown that the adoption process for an agricultural technology, be it seeds or fertilizer, follows a typical "S"-shaped curve. After a new technological advance is introduced, the first farmers to adopt it are taking a grave economic risk. For example, if hybrid corn (Figure 10.1) had failed when it was introduced in the 1930's, those farmers who first tried it would have taken a severe loss in crops and income. Because hybrid corn was successful, those who adopted it first reaped the greatest

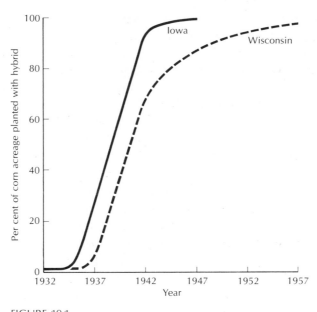

FIGURE 10.1.
Cycle of adoption for hybrid corn in the U.S. (From Z. Griliches, "Hybrid Corn: An Exploration in the Economics of Technological Change," Econometrica, Oct. 1957, 502.)

economic rewards. They had the highest yields, and the increase in income more than offset the price of the seedcorn they had to buy from the corn breeders. New technologies are often adopted first on the biggest and most prosperous farms, for these are managed by farmers who keep abreast of the new developments in agriculture and have the capital needed to profit from such developments. The later a farmer adopted hybrid corn, the less would be his relative economic benefit. The last farmers to adopt it did so out of necessity: it became hard to run a profitable farming operation without hybrid corn. It should be noted that the ultimate benefits of this adoption cycle were increased corn production and a relatively lower price for the consumers.

Mexico

The case of wheat in Mexico represents the only example of a completed adoption cycle for one of the high-yielding cereal grains that form the basis of the green revolution. The Mexican government embarked on a program to increase wheat production not because the people were hungry or the farmers were poor, but because wheat imports were so expensive that the country was being drained of its foreign currency reserves. Self-sufficiency in wheat would reduce this drain on the Mexican economy, and make it possible to lower the price consumers paid for wheat products. In partnership with the Rockefeller Foundation, the Mexican government set up the breeding stations which developed the semidwarf wheats. These wheat strains were then planted throughout Mexico.

The adoption curve for high-yielding wheat in Mexico again follows the typical "S" shape; completion of the entire cycle took about a dozen years (Figure 10.2). By 1954, when the wheat adoption cycle was five years old, half of the entire Mexican wheat acreage was planted with the new varieties, and over-all wheat yields were up about 50 percent from those of five years before. By 1959, with the cycle ten years old, wheat yields had doubled, and the country was becoming self-sufficient in wheat. Also, about 90 percent of the wheat acreage was planted with the new strains. Finally, in 1964, fifteen years after the initial plantings of the new strains, Mexico began exporting wheat. In the meantime, as wheat production went up, prices fell, and by 1964 the price of wheat in Mexico was half of what it had been a decade before. Clearly, this aspect of the green revolution in Mexico had succeeded in reaching its objectives.

Asia

In Asia, the primary objective of the green revolution is to improve the diets of an increasing and ill-fed population. An additional objective, similar to the one pursued by Mexico, was to reduce currency losses from imports. In a position paper presented at the 1974 World Food Conference, the F.A.O. estimated that, given their current levels of agricultural production, the underdeveloped countries would need to import 85 million tons of cereal grains per year by 1985. Current (1976) import levels are about 35 million tons. The estimated cost of such an import, based on a conservative price of $200 per ton, is $16–$18 billion per year. This would be an intolerable drain on the economies of the underdeveloped countries. Thus, they must improve their own capacity to produce food.

The adoption cycle for high-yielding wheat and rice has been underway in Asia since the late 1960's. Acreages planted with the new varieties have increased every year, and are still increasing (see Table 10.1). When these acreages are expressed as percentages of the available area (see Figure

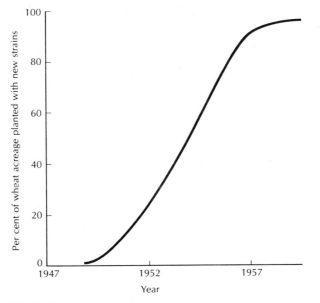

FIGURE 10.2.
Cycles of adoption for high-yielding wheat in Mexico.
(From D. Dalrymple, Economic Research Service, U.S.D.A.)

Table 10.1 Acreage planted in high-yielding wheat and rice in Asia (excluding China), in thousands of acres.[a]

Year	Wheat	Rice
1965–1966	23	18
1966–1967	1,542	2,505
1967–1968	10,189	6,847
1968–1969	19,815	11,620
1969–1970	21,550	19,104
1970–1971	27,211	25,207
1971–1972	33,353	33,218
1972–1973	39,097	38,692
1973–1974	43,000	41,000
1974–1975	49,000	46,000

[a]From "Development and spread of high-yielding varieties of wheat and rice in less developed nations" (U.S.D.A. 1974), and other U.S.D.A. data.

10.3), the Asian green revolution can be seen to be at the midpoint in the adoption cycle. Massive economic supports by several Asian governments initially speeded up the usual adoption process, and the adoption rate is now beginning to slow down. However, if a reasonable expansion of the new varieties onto new lands continues, all of the wheat acreage in the Indian subcontinent will be planted with high-yielding varieties by the 1980's.

A comparison of the increase in wheat yields obtained in Asia with that obtained in Mexico (Figure 10.4) also indicates that the green revolution is at the midpont of its cycle in the Asian countries. There has been a steady rise in over-all wheat yield since the new seed varieties were introduced. The situation is similar for those countries where high-yielding rice has been planted. Trends toward an increased over-all yield have been observed in all countries as the use of high-yielding varieties has increased. Indeed, in a 1973 survey, the International Rice Research Institute found

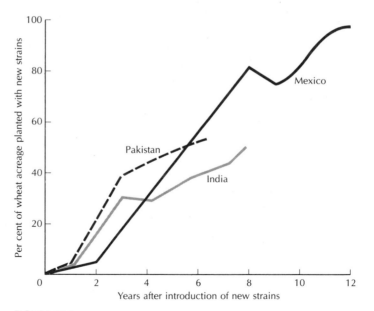

FIGURE 10.3.
Cycles of adoption for high-yielding varieties of wheat. The year of initial adoption (year "zero") was 1947–1948 for Mexico, 1966–1967 for India, and 1967–1968 for Pakistan. (From D. Dalrymple, U.S.D.A.)

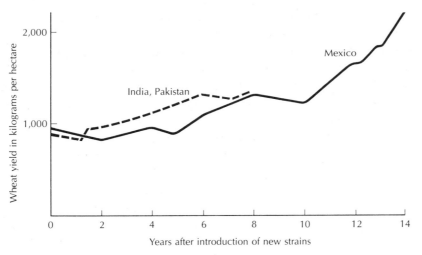

FIGURE 10.4.
Wheat yields (national) during the adoption cycle for high-yielding wheat. (From D. Dalrymple, U.S.D.A.)

that the percentage increase in national rice yield from 1961–1971 corresponded almost exactly with the percentage of land converted to the new strains. For example, rice yields increased by 50 percent in the Philippines, and 56 percent of the land had been planted with IR-5 and IR-8 strains.

In spite of the increases in yields reportedly due to the new strains, these increases are certainly far below those predicted from experimental plots at agricultural research stations. When the Asian green revolution began, available data indicated that the high-yielding strains could produce five times as much grain per acre per year as their counterparts then in use. In actual practice in the fields and paddies of Asia, the new wheats have produced a yield 2.5 to 3.0 times that of traditional varieties, and the new rices have a yield multiple of about 2.0. These numbers, obtained from the U.S.D.A., are high, and reflect the fact that so far only the best land in Asia has been used for the new varieties. Further expansion of the new varieties will be on less productive soils. If land quality is equalized, Dr. D. Dalrymple of the U.S.D.A. estimates that in irrigated areas the high-yielding wheats might yield 2.0 times more grain than the traditional strains. The yield multiple for rice can be expected to be around 1.25.

Although it is unreasonable to expect farmers to duplicate the results obtained in experiment stations, the gap between the potential and the actual yields of the high-yielding strains is a cause for concern. To discover the reasons for this gap, the International Rice Research Institute in 1973 surveyed 15 rice farms in Laguna province in the Philippines. The small farmers in this survey were all using the high-yielding varieties, but obtaining a yield multiple of only 1.5 times that of the traditional varieties. By comparison, experimental plots at the Institute, also in the Philippines, reported yield multiples of 3.5 and 4.0 for the same rice strains. There were three causes for the shortfall on the farms: inadequate water, inadequate nitrogen fertilizer, and diseases. These three factors are the major constraints on both area and yield expansion of the Asian green revolution.

CONSTRAINTS ON EXPANSION

Water

The inability of the farmers to meet the water requirements of the crops and to control the flow of water is the most significant factor preventing the expansion of the acreage used for the high-yielding varieties. Indeed, this inability is a major reason why, as of the mid-1970's, the green revolution for wheat has been limited to southern and western Asia and for rice to southern and eastern Asia. Even within these broad areas there are significant regional differences: in 1973, 74 percent of the high-yield wheat in Pakistan was grown in one province and 77 percent of the rice in another province. Inadequate control over the supply and the flow of water makes it impossible to grow these strains in most of the other areas. It has been predicted that inadequate water control will mean that the acreage adoption cycles for the new wheat and rice strains will never reach 100 percent.

On the average, rice requires about three times as much water per acre as wheat. Not only does rice require large amounts of water, but it must also receive the water at a particular time during development. An important genetic property of the high-yielding rice strains is their high capacity to send out extra seed-bearing stems called tillers. Studies in the Philippines have shown that tillering is greater in shallow water than in deep water. Thus if too much water is provided during this developmental stage, crop yield is reduced. Later, during the period of grain swelling, the plant is very sensitive to too little water. Likewise, wheat is sensitive to dry conditions throughout its growth, and lack of water seriously reduces yields. A controllable water supply is not ensured if one depends on the weather, and for this reason the new strains have not been used widely in the monsoon regions of Asia.

Irrigation provides water control, and it is on irrigated lands such as those in the Indo-Gangetic plain that the high-yielding cereal strains have performed best. In Asia as of the mid-1970's, irrigated land represented 20 percent of the cultivated acreage and provided 40 percent of the food production. Rainfed land without water control accounted for 60 percent of the cultivated area and produced half the food. The remaining land, in upland areas, contributed 10 percent of the food. A study carried out in the Philippines in 1970 clearly showed the difference between rice yields obtained on irrigated land and those obtained on rainfed land (Table 10.2).

To overcome the fact that water control limits the expansion of acreage planted with the high-yielding varieties, two kinds of corrective measures have been tried. The first approach is to breed plants better adapted to the climatic conditions prevailing in these areas. In Mexico, strains of high-yielding wheat are being developed which show an increased tolerance to dry conditions. The wheat-rye hybrid Triticale is especially promising in this regard. Rice strains are being bred which are high-yielding but less sensitive to water stress than are the strains currently in use. The second approach is a broad water-management program. Irrigation in Asia comes from canals (40 percent) and tubewells (30 percent). Many canal systems are poorly constructed and have considerable seepage, which causes the irrigation water to be too salty. This problem can be corrected by either relining the canals or speeding up the flow of water so that seepage is negligible. But even with a massive program of water control, it is doubtful that the high-yielding varieties will spread to cover all of Asia.

In Africa, the water situation is worse. Most African rivers dry up in the dry season, and, when the rain comes, flooding and soil erosion are

Table 10.2. Water supply and rice production in the Philippines, 1970.[a]

Conditions	Per cent of crop as high-yielding varieties	Yield in tons per hectare
Fully irrigated	96.5	2.7
Partly irrigated	62.5	2.1
Rainfed	31.6	1.8

[a]From I.R.R.I. data.

common. Thus much of Africa is unsuitable for irrigation; for example, the F.A.O. has estimated that only 2 percent of the land in Tanzania is suitable for irrigation. Extension of the green revolution into many parts of Africa must await the development of new crop strains which are not only high-yielding but also resistant to water stress.

Soil problems, often related to water problems, are a serious constraint on the spread of the high-yielding cereal varieties. Salinity, a problem in lowland deltas, estuaries, and some irrigated regions, has affected over 30 million hectares in Asia and Africa, rendering them unsuitable for the growth of the new strains of wheat and rice. Alkalinity is a problem in about 4 million hectares of the arid regions of India, Pakistan, and the Middle East. This can be overcome by applying gypsum to the soil to neutralize the alkalinity, followed by irrigation. However, this soil-reclamation process is quite expensive. Zinc deficiency, common in lowland soils, and iron toxicity, common in the highly weathered soils of the humid tropics, are currently under intensive study in order to develop crop strains which can produce high yields under these conditions.

Technological Inputs

The 1973–1974 "energy crisis" dramatically demonstrated that both the green revolution and agricultural production in technologically advanced countries are dependent on fossil fuels and other technological inputs. The new crop strains cannot produce high yields if irrigation pumps, the necessary fuel to run them, farm machinery, pesticides, and fertilizers are lacking. The manufacture of these technological inputs requires large amounts of energy. The new crop strains produce larger grain crops but use more nutrients from the soil, and these nutrients must be replaced by means of fertilizer added to the soil. When no fertilizer is added, the new strains of wheat and rice still produce somewhat higher yields than the traditional varieties. However, the differences in yield between the two types of strains are much more pronounced when the soil is fertilized (see Figure 10.5). We saw in Chapter 7 that nearly a third of the energy needed to produce corn in the U.S.A. is used to manufacture nitrogen fertilizers (industrial nitrogen fixation). Thus, fertilizer production is also an agricultural input which requires large amounts of energy.

Surveys of fertilizer use in the Philippines and India have consistently shown that farmers use too little fertilizer to meet the demands of the high-

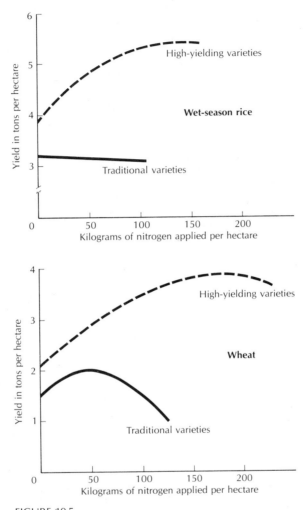

FIGURE 10.5.
*Fertilizer-response curves for rice and wheat varieties in
Asia. (Data from U.S.D.A. and I.R.R.I.)*

yielding strains. The reason for this is economic: most small farmers cannot
afford the needed supplies of fertilizer, especially since prices have risen
steeply during the last decade. As energy becomes scarce and costly, fertilizer is becoming less available to the underdeveloped nations. It is not
surprising, then, that the Indian government in late 1974 called for a massive

switch from synthetic inorganic fertilizer to organic fertilizer derived from human and animal wastes.

The availability and cost of fuel has seriously threatened the green revolution. Fuel is needed to run irrigation pumps, planters, and harvesters. Although some of these functions can be replaced by human labor, often they cannot be, at least not without a loss in yield and in over-all production. During the Arab oil embargo of 1973–1974, diesel fuel needed to run irrigation pumps became so scarce that farmers in India lined up for days to get a few gallons of fuel. The current high price of fuel is clearly an impediment to the further spread and maximum use of the high-yielding varieties.

The demand for pesticides has increased at about 20 percent per year (F.A.O. 1974 estimate), but production has remained more or less constant. As a result, pesticide prices have increased, and the poor farmers who are planting high-yielding wheat and rice have been using less pesticide. Since pests were already destroying a significant portion of the crop, this situation has led to a considerable reduction in potential yield. Although progress has been made in breeding of pest-resistant crop strains, the F.A.O. recommends that current pesticide use in the underdeveloped regions should be at least doubled.

Clearly, massive increases in agricultural technologies are needed to maximize the potential of the green revolution in food production. But what would be the effects of such an assault on the natural environment? Would massive doses of chemical fertilizers lead to poisoning of the drinking water, eutrophication of fresh inland waters, and irreversible increases in salinity? Would increased use of pesticides lead to the deaths of other, non-pest organisms, including man? A number of ecologists, such as G. Hardin of the University of California, feel that the point of maximum despoilation of the environment has been reached, and that any further increases in use of fertilizers or pesticides, for example, will lead to a global disaster. The Earth, say these ecologists, is a "commons" whose resources, food-production capacity, and ability to absorb pollutants are finite and now in maximum use. Any attempt to increase food production by current agricultural practice will, in their opinion, irreversibly upset the balance of nature. Most agriculturalists are not convinced that this view is correct. They feel that food-production possibilities can and should be maximized, and that ways must be found to increase crop production without upsetting the balance of nature.

SOCIAL AND ECONOMIC IMPACT

Local Effects

When the green revolution began in Asia, economists and sociologists predicted that it would exacerbate the gap between rich and poor farmers in this region. This prediction has indeed come true. In Asia, as in many other parts of the world, there are many more small landowners and landless farmers than there are large landowners. For example, in the Punjab region of Pakistan, 21 percent of the farmers cultivate 68 percent of the land, most of it in holdings of four hectares or more, but the remaining 79 percent of the farmers farm only 32 percent of the land, in holdings of less than four hectares. Most of the larger farmers own their farms, whereas the small farmers are either sharecroppers who give a fixed proportion of their harvest to the owner or renters who pay a fixed rent to the owner. In return for providing their landlords with cheap labor, the sharecroppers would also receive a fixed proportion of the harvest. In good years, they would share in the bounty; in lean years, the landlords would give them an extra share of the crop to enable them to survive.

The introduction of the green revolution into Asia has upset these traditional arrangements in several ways. We stressed earlier that the yield potential of the new strains of wheat and rice can only be reached if the necessary technological inputs, such as water, fertilizer, and pesticides, are provided. Small farmers, generally, tend to minimize their risks. They must spend a great deal of their income on food and other necessities, and have little capital to buy the technological inputs necessary for high-yield agriculture. The wealthier Asian farmers did possess the necessary capital to invest in seeds, irrigation equipment, and fertilizers, and consequently they profited from the green revolution. Furthermore, government policies did not include financial assistance to poorer farmers to help them make the necessary purchases.

In the industrialized nations, as technological innovations were adopted in the agricultural sector, many of the poorer farmers with small farms were forced to sell their farms, being unable to maintain an adequate living standard. They migrated to the cities and joined the new industrial work force there. The underdeveloped countries have hoped to accomplish the same result by means of the green revolution. They hoped that the development of large, mechanized farms would increase food production and hold food costs down, would thus help transfer economic wealth from the agricultural sector to the industrial sector, and would create a labor force from the landless farmers. In Mexico this strategy has been partly successful, because the government's policy is to create half a million new jobs each year. Unfortunately, 800,000 new job seekers are added to the labor force each year. In Asia this strategy has not worked at all. There are simply too many people to be absorbed even by a growing industrial base. Migration from the countryside has only resulted in overcrowded cities with high unemployment and extreme poverty.

The green revolution has also upset the paternalistic relationship between sharecropper and landowner. In a study of Pakistan and India, sociologist Francine Frankel found that, when harvests increased dramatically, the landowner no longer wished to pay his harvesters with a fixed proportion of the harvest. Rather, the same amount of the grain harvest was given to the laborers as had been given in previous years. Moreover, the landlord no longer felt an obligation toward landless laborers. In the past, these people would be allowed to share in a good harvest to build up their stocks of food. Now, with harvests booming, the landowner could contract with an outside buyer to sell his excess production. Thus the green revolution in Asia has allowed the rich to become richer and the poor to remain poor.

Can the small farmers benefit from the green revolution, and should the government encourage small farmers to stay on the land? It is generally true that large farming operations tend to be capital-intensive, whereas small farmers are much more labor-intensive. Human labor is the most important input in the small farms in Taiwan, where the practices of inter-cropping and relay cropping allow the farmers to grow six or more crops each year on the same piece of land. These farmers cannot afford to buy the technological inputs needed to get maximum yields from the new strains. As the prices of these inputs rise—and they rose significantly in the early 1970's—it becomes less likely that the small farmers will be able to afford any fertilizer or pesticides. However, there is much evidence which suggests that the farmers on the small, labor-intensive farms can get a higher yield from the same crop strain than those who operate the larger, capital-intensive farms. For example, a study by economist Keith Griffin of farm size, capital intensity, and yield of rice in Ceylon (Table 10.3) showed that yields on the smallest farms with the least technological inputs were approximately 10 percent higher than those on the larger farms. The reasons for this phenomenon are not entirely clear, but it is well-known that the operators of

Table 10.3. Farm size, capital intensity, and yield of rice in Ceylon, 1967.[a]

Farm size, in perches[b]	Labor cost[c]	Seed sown, in bushels per acre	Tractor cost[c]	Herbicide cost[c]	Fertilizer, in pounds per acre	Capital intensity index	Yield, in bushels per acre
0–20	428	2.57	18.5	1.65	107	100	37.4
21–40	405	2.29	18.7	4.25	118	120	37.3
41–80	335	2.24	19.3	2.36	129	137	33.6
81–160	259	2.30	21.1	2.12	112	190	31.8
161–320	204	2.22	42.4	3.64	77	479	33.0
More than 320	180	2.56	65.2	5.22	157	833	33.7
Average	212	2.45	51.3	4.34	136	—	33.5

[a]From K. Griffin, *The Green Revolution: An Economic Analysis* (U.N. Res. Inst. Social Development, 1972), p. 36.

[b]A perch is about 30 square yards.

[c]In rupees per acre.

very small farms take extremely good care of their crops. The data indicate that spreading the green revolution to the small farmers will be beneficial in terms of food production, as well as in terms of economics and sociology. Encouraging the small farmers to stay on the land and making available to them some of the inputs of the green revolution (especially higher-yielding, disease-resistant strains) will increase food production without the social dislocations caused by the movements of millions of people from the land to the cities.

Several projects are underway that attempt to reach the small farmer. One of the most successful is the Puebla project, 75 miles east of Mexico City. In 1967, small teams of agricultural extension workers were sent out into the small farms of the region with two objectives: to convince the farmers that new strains of corn were a risk worth taking; and to convince local bankers that the small farmers were worthy of credit, so that they could purchase the new seeds and their associated technologies. Local groups were set up, and by 1971 there were 183 such groups with 5,240 participating farmers. The groups were able to obtain credit, as a group, that they could never have obtained as individuals. Under the direction of an extension worker, each group set up a small demonstration plot of the new seeds with fertilizer and irrigation, on one farm. Once the other farmers in the group saw the results of the demonstration, they immediately chose to adopt the new technology. The result is that farmers whose average yield was 16 bushels of corn per acre in 1967 now report yields of over 80 bushels per acre.

The two key aspects of the success of the Puebla project, agriculturalists working directly with the farmers and credit availability, are being used elsewhere. In India, the agriculture department has steadily lowered the minimum farm size for credit availability. In 1966, credit was given only to farmers with more than 20 acres; in 1967, the minimum was 15 acres; in 1970, the minimum was two acres. New land-ownership laws in India make large holdings illegal, and a redistribution of land to the poor is beginning. However, as the land is redistributed, it becomes imperative that the poor have access to the improved means of food production. If they do not, production will be reduced significantly.

Global Agriculture

Our modern world is characterized by interdependence in many areas. Bumper crops or crop failures in one part of the world have an impact on food prices and food reserves in the whole world. The recent history of grain production and agricultural policy in the U.S.S.R. illustrates well the truly global nature of agriculture and food production. Grain production in the U.S.S.R. has shown an upward trend since 1960 (Figure 10.6). However, there have been large fluctuations from year to year, because fully two-thirds of the U.S.S.R. grain crop is produced north of the 49th parallel, where rainfall is not dependable. In 1972 insufficient rainfall and harsh winter weather cut the Russian wheat crop by over 10 million tons. When the U.S.S.R. experienced grain shortfalls in 1963, 1965, and 1967, it dealt with the situation by remaining self-sufficient and simply consuming less grain for those years. In 1970, however, the government embarked on a plan to increase meat consumption as a symbol of affluence and nutritional improvement. Thus, from 1966 to 1974, cereal-grain consumption per capita in the U.S.S.R. rose by 30 percent, with most of this rise resulting from increased use of feed grains. In 1972, Russia suffered another poor grain harvest. However, rather than cut meat consumption, the government

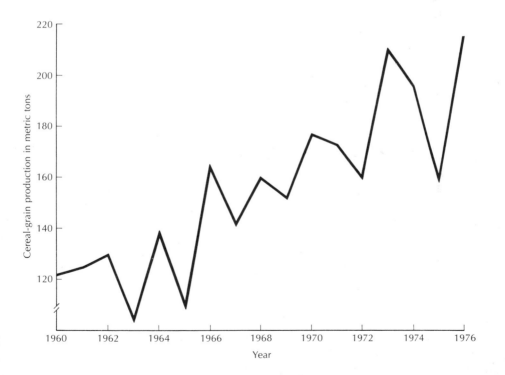

FIGURE 10.6.
Grain production in the U.S.S.R. (Data from U.S.D.A.)

made up the difference between needed and actual grain on hand by massive imports. Within a few months, the U.S.S.R. purchased 28 million tons of grain on the world market, including 18 million tons from the U.S. This reduced the available grain on the world market, and prices rose dramatically.

In 1972, several other factors also had an impact on world food supplies. Droughts in Argentina and Australia cut their grain production. A subnormal monsoon in India reduced the wheat crop for the first time since the beginning of the green revolution there. An excessively wet autumn delayed and reduced the U.S. corn and bean harvests. The catch of Peruvian anchovies, a major source of feed protein, plummeted, causing additional demand for feed grains. Finally, rising affluence in Europe was causing an increase in the demand for and consumption of meat, and placed an extra burden on the feed-grain supply. In combination, these factors had two effects: a doubling in the prices of wheat, rice, corn, and soybeans from 1972 to 1973, and a severe reduction in stored reserves of grain (see Figure 10.7).

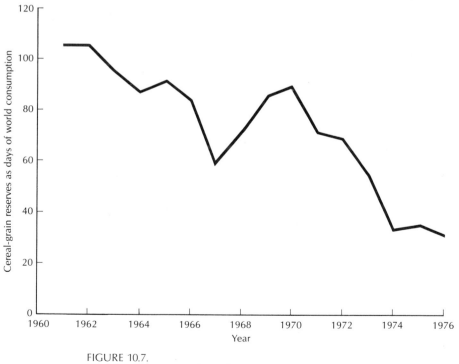

FIGURE 10.7.
World grain reserves. (Data from U.S.D.A. and the F.A.O.)

The reduction in grain reserves raised serious alarms, and was a major reason for the holding of a World Food Conference in 1974. People have realized since ancient times the need to store grain for later use in case of a bad harvest. The U.N., at the Food Conference, estimated that the cost of keeping a reasonable amount of stored grain (20 percent of world consumption, equal to the greatest recent shortfall of grain) would be about $1 billion per year, with an initial investment of $5 billion. The problem of who should pay for this "food insurance" has led to an examination of the role of food aid in the global economics of agriculture.

In the past, the United States has been an important supplier of food aid to many underdeveloped countries. Massive agricultural aid by the U.S. began in 1954 with the passage of Public Law 480, "an act to increase consumption of U.S. agricultural commodities in foreign countries, to improve the foreign relations of the U.S., and for other purposes." The purposes of the food shipments were economic and political, not primarily humanitarian. Between 1955 and 1970, some $16.2 billion in food sold at low prices to poor countries brought the U.S. foreign exchange and political friends in the recipient countries. It allowed the American farmers to earn extra income which would otherwise have been lost, since the recipient countries were unable to buy the food at world market prices. In the 1973 report on Public Law 480 prepared by the U.S.D.A. for the U.S. Congress, the strategic and political importance of food aid was emphasized: most aid in that year went to South Korea, Vietnam, Israel, Pakistan, and Indonesia. Although it is certainly true that U.S. food aid has served a valuable humanitarian purpose—massive shipments in 1966 averted disaster in India—the main goals of the aid had been concerned with economics and foreign policy. After the World Food Conference in 1974, the U.S. in 1975 more than doubled its food aid to the poorest countries, and passed a law that 70 percent of the aid must go to those countries regarded as most affected by adverse world economic conditions. Nevertheless, these countries still purchase much of their grain on the world market and at market prices. With grain surpluses dwindling or nonexistent, there is little economic incentive for the U.S. to ship food to poor countries when it can receive the full price for grain from affluent countries. In 1975, in the midst of another grain shortfall in the U.S.S.R. (Figure 10.6), the U.S. signed long-term agreements for grain exports to several countries, including Japan and the U.S.S.R.

These pressures on the world agricultural system make progress in the green revolution more urgent than ever before. If there are no massive shipments of American grain during the next Indian drought, it is clear that India will have to have her own stocks of grain in order to survive. If the cost of importing grain into Asia is becoming intolerable, it is clear that Asia must become self-sufficient in grain production. Aid should now be in the form of investments or loans to improve local agriculture, rather than outright gifts of food. The World Bank has been especially active in this regard. The F.A.O. has estimated that about 50 billion dollars are needed by the underdeveloped countries if they are to double their agricultural production by 1985.

NUTRITIONAL IMPACT

The emphasis in the Asian green revolution has been on the production of more food, not on production of nutritionally better food. Because surplus crops can be sold on the world market, many countries have begun growing the high-yielding cereal grains on lands previously used for growing protein-rich legumes. Although cereal-grain yields have been increased by the green revolution, yields of legumes have not (see Table 10.4). As a result, the over-all diet of their populations has shifted from a mixture of cereals and legumes to one emphasizing cereals. As we pointed out in Chapter 3, such a diet can lead to protein malnutrition. This trend away from legumes was also observed during the early years of the Mexican green revolution, but

Table 10.4. Annual wheat, rice, and legume productions, in thousands of metric tons.[a]

	1948–1952 (average)	1961–1965 (average)	1966	1970	1974
Mexico:					
Wheat	534	1,537	1,612	2,100	2,300
Dry beans	235	761	1,002	1,300	1,350
India:					
Rice		52,760	45,657	62,500	59,500
Wheat		11,198	10,424	20,093	24,700
Groundnuts		5,095	4,411	6,100	5,800
Indonesia:					
Rice		12,719	14,009	16,839	23,538
Soybeans		395	417	408	550

[a]Data from F.A.O. Production Yearbooks.

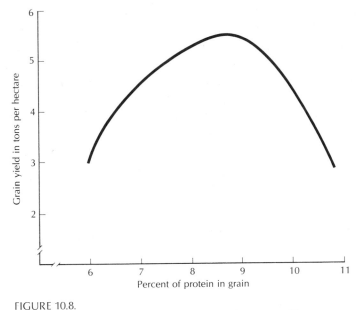

FIGURE 10.8.
Protein content and yield of IR-8 rice, 1973 dry season. (From I.R.R.I. Research Highlights, 1973, p. 23.)

once Mexico was self-sufficient in wheat, the production of legumes began to rise. Hopefully, the Mexican example will be followed in Asia.

The economics of world trade consistently ignores nutrition. Africa exports legumes and groundnuts when its people are suffering from protein malnutrition. Asia and the Far East in 1972 exported 5 percent of their legume production. Latin America exports about 15 percent of its meat production and an equal percentage of its corn crop. The recipients of this protein are the affluent, whose diets are already excessive in protein. With the foreign exchange they receive for exporting protein, the underdeveloped countries often buy carbohydrate-rich cereals.

High-yielding wheat and rice strains were bred for yield, and little attention was paid to the nutritional value of the grain (e.g., its protein content). Increases in yield above a certain level are accompanied by a decrease in the protein content of the grain (see Figure 10.8). This phenomenon has also been noted in the U.S.A., where higher yields of wheat have resulted in a decreased protein content of the grain. Thus the maximal yield produces a crop with a lower protein content and hence a lower nutritional value. Plant breeders have shown that this problem can be corrected by selecting strains whose response to nitrogen fertilizers is to increase their seed-protein production and to produce high yields at the same time. At the International Rice Research Institute a new rice strain, IR 480-5-9, has an optimum yield of 16 tons per acre with a protein content at that yield of 10.3 percent. High-protein, high-lysine wheat strains developed by the U.S.D.A. in Nebraska are being crossed with high-yielding varieties to produce more nutritious wheat. Finally, a major effort has begun in the U.S. and India to improve the yield of legumes. These research projects are for the future. For now, the green revolution has meant averting starvation for millions, but their over-all diet has not improved in quality.

CHAPTER 11 Alternative Sources of Food

Most human food is produced by traditional crop agriculture, which is the most obvious method, since most human calories and protein come directly from plants. However, traditional agriculture has biological and environmental limits, and if the human population continues to increase, these limits will soon be reached. This situation gives impetus to the search for alternative sources of food.

FOOD FROM THE SEA

The ocean has long been considered the potential panacea for the food demands of the future. After all, the argument goes, sea waters cover 70 percent of the earth's surface, and endless resources must abound in so vast an area.

The present oceanic catch contributes only 1 percent of the calories and 10 percent of the protein to the human diet, and it was thought that these figures could be greatly increased simply by intensification of the fishing* technology that is now in use.

In 1938, the total world fish catch was 20 million tons; by 1968, it had passed 60 million tons. A major reason for this increase was the technological modernization of fishing fleets. The fishing fleets of such nations as the U.S.S.R., and Japan, and the U.S. have expanded greatly since 1940. Russia

---

*The term "fishing" is used here to cover all activities which result in obtaining food from the sea. It includes hunting sea mammals, such as whales, as well as catching shrimp, lobsters, krill, and other arthropods, and gathering clams, mussels, and other mollusks.

was the first to use factory ships, floating cities that accommodate over 10,000 people and are equipped with processing facilities for freezing, salting, canning, and preserving fish on the spot. Fish schools are located by sonar and Earth satellites, and the fish are caught with improved gear, such as trawls, traps, and seines. Those who hope to increase the food that people obtain from the sea often make claims similar to those of green-revolution proponents: more technology will mean more food.

However, unlike agriculture, where man controls the environment to grow food, fishing is essentially a form of hunting. As a result, the fish catch is limited by the oceanic productivity. The primary producers of the oceanic food chain are microscopic green plants, the phytoplankton. Like their counterparts, these plants require sunlight, carbon dioxide, oxygen, and minerals in order to grow and reproduce. Sunlight and dissolved gases are abundant in surface waters. However the supply of minerals may be inadequate at the surface, especially in the open ocean. Since most minerals settle on the bottom, mineral concentrations at the surface of deep waters will be low unless some mechanism brings the minerals to the surface. In nontropical oceans, such as the North Atlantic and Southern Oceans, waters are mixed by the alternate warming and cooling during the changing seasons. This mixing brings some minerals to the surface of deep waters. However, in the tropical oceans, such mixing does not occur. Because minerals are scarce, phytoplankton growth is minimal, and the open ocean, especially in the tropics, has a low primary productivity.

In two areas of the ocean, mineral concentrations in surface waters are adequate for abundant phytoplankton growth. The first is the shallow coastal zone (180 meters or less in depth), where runoff from rivers constantly supplies an abundance of minerals. The second comprises regions of coastal upwelling. These regions occur off the coasts of Peru, California, and parts of Africa, where there are seasonal offshore winds and currents. Surface waters are diverted offshore and replaced with mineral-rich deeper water. Together, the coastal and upwelling regions occupy only 10 percent of the oceanic surface; but they supply more than 95 percent of the food people derive from the sea.

The fish eaten by human beings are generally those at the top of the marine food chain. In upwelling areas, there may be only one or two intermediate organisms from the primary producers, the phytoplankton, to the human consumer. But in the coastal zone or open sea, marine food chains may include six or seven different species. Oceanographer J. Ryther has estimated that the efficiencies of energy transfer (Chapter 4) between the levels of the food chains are 10 percent, 15 percent, and 20 percent for the open oceanic, coastal, and upwelling areas, respectively. Using these estimates, as well as values assigned to the three areas for primary productivity, Ryther has estimated the total annual fish production in the three regions (Table 11.1). Some 90 percent of the oceanic surface is, for fishing, a biological desert, with most of the fish being in the coastal and upwelling zones. The total annual fish production, about 250 million tons, is approximately four times the present annual fish catch. Unfortunately, production is not equivalent to potential harvest. People must be careful to leave a large-enough fraction of the annual production of fish to reproduce, so that the fish catch can be sustained year after year. In addition, people must take into account that other carnivores, especially birds and mammals, consume fish. With these limiting factors in mind, the maximum sustainable fish catch is about 120 million tons per year, about twice the present catch. This figure assumes an intelligent exploitation of the resources of the ocean. Recent trends toward overfishing and oceanic pollution indicate that the maximum sustainable yield may be significantly reduced.

Increasing demand for fish and meat (about a fourth of the fish catch is processed into fishmeal and used for livestock feed) has led to an increasing competition for the world's annual fish production. Such is the demand for more fish that coastal zones have become regions of hot dispute among fishing nations. At the 1973 and 1975 "Law of the Sea" conferences spon-

Table 11.1. Productivity of the sea.[a]

	Open ocean	Coastal zone	Upwelling zone
Percent of ocean	90	9.9	0.1
Productivity (grams of CO_2 fixed per square meter per year)	50	100	300
Total productivity (billions of tons of carbon per year)	16.3	3.6	0.1
Trophic levels	5	3	2
Fish production (in millions of tons)	2–4	100–200	100–200

[a]From J. Ryther, "Photosynthesis and Fish Production in the Sea," *Science*, 166 (1969), 73. Copyright 1969 by the American Association for the Advancement of Science.

sored by the U.N., most fishing nations took the attitude that they owned the coastal waters of their own countries up to 200 miles offshore, but that the waters off *other* countries should be available to all! This competition has also led to overfishing and the eventual depletion of stocks of several fish, including the sardines in the waters off California and the herring off Japan.

The most recent and dramatic example of what can happen to an over-fished population is provided by the anchovy. These fish congregate in the cool coastal currents off the coast of Peru. During the summer, these regions are very narrow and the anchovies pack together in this restrictedd zone. Dozens of tons of them can be taken in this zone at one time; so it is not surprising that, from a modest beginning in the 1950's, the anchovy catch rose to over 10 million tons a year in the late 1960's. This amount was greater than that of all other fish caught by all Western nations combined. The fishmeal made from the Peruvian anchovies is exported as livestock feed; the oil goes into margarine, paint, and even lipstick.

In 1972, the anchovy catch plummeted to 4 million tons (Figure 11.1), a disaster for the Peruvian economy. Why did it occur? First, because the coastal waters had warmed up, and this lowered the anchovies' survival and reproduction. Second, biologists had warned that, to ensure survival of the anchovy during these climatic changes, which occur regularly near Peru, the annual catch should not exceed 10 million tons per year. This limit had been exceeded in the two years before the 1972 disaster. Biologists are uncertain whether the anchovy population will ever recover.

Pollution may seriously reduce the potential productivity of the oceans. The primary productivity of the North Atlantic has declined by 20 percent since 1950. This decline may be a natural cyclic variation, or it may be caused by pollution. Many chemicals, waste products of a technological society, are being dumped into the rivers and end up in the ocean, or are dumped directly into the oceans. Oil slicks from offshore oil wells, tanker accidents, tanker cleaning operations, or natural seepage through the ocean floor, which has been observed in the open ocean, all have an *unknown* effect on ocean productivity. Residues of pesticides, especially DDT and other chlorinated hydrocarbons, have been found in the oceans, especially in the coastal waters, which are rich in fish. When several species of marine algae were grown in the laboratory, it was found that their photosynthesis was inhibited by minute amounts (a few thousandths of a milligram per liter) of DDT. It is fortunate that the amount of chlorinated hydrocarbons in the

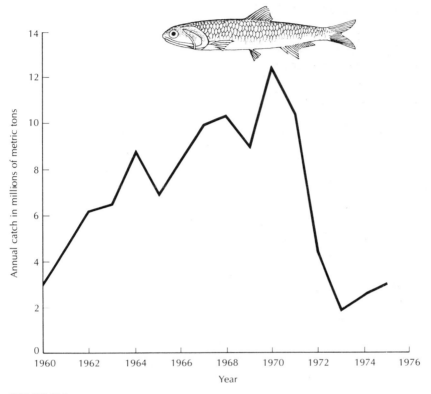

FIGURE 11.1.
The worldwide anchovy catch, 1955–1973. (Adapted from C. Idyll, "The Anchovy." Copyright © 1973 by Scientific American, Inc. All rights reserved.)

oceans has probably not yet reached these inhibitory concentrations. In fresh waters, dangerous levels of mercury have been found in many rivers and lakes, and this toxic metal has, via the food chain, found its way into fish, making them unfit for human consumption. In some areas, pollution by toxic chemicals has caused huge fish kills. Whether such occurrences will be common in oceanic fisheries is unknown, but it is now obvious that industrialized nations cannot continue to "dispose" of their dangerous and unwanted chemicals in the oceans without seriously jeopardizing the oceans' food-producing capacity.

AQUACULTURE

People fish by hunting. On land, hunting was largely abandoned when agriculture began (Chapter 6). Some scientists propose that food procurement from the sea will undergo a similar transition, and that *aquaculture,* the cultivation of marine organisms, will soon be practiced on a large scale.

Aquaculture is not new. It was common over 4,000 years ago in China, Japan, and Egypt. Currently it supplies about 4 percent of the global fish harvest, but could supply much more. The most successful aquaculture systems do not rear the organisms in an enclosed environment for their entire life cycle. Rather, the young are captured and reared to maturity in ponds adjacent to the sea. Within these areas, nutrients may be supplied (a "fertilizer" input), and predators are kept away. Oysters, mussels, and shrimp are raised in this way.

Oyster culture provides an example of highly successful aquaculture. Oysters normally live in shallow water, attached to various hard objects on the bottom. They feed by filtering plankton and other organic matter from the water. When a single oyster spawns, it produces more than 100 million eggs, which hatch into free-swimming immature oysters (larvae). After two to three weeks, these larvae attach themselves to hard surfaces and, in a few years, become full-sized oysters. For oyster cultivation, an area along the coast is fenced off and all predators, especially starfish, within the enclosure are removed. Smooth, hard surfaces, such as ceramic tiles, are placed on the sea bottom to ensure proper spacing. Another method is used in Japan, where the oysters develop on long strings hanging from floats. The oysters not only are protected from predators, but also receive an excellent diet, because the tidal flow brings in a great deal of food. This method of oyster culture has produced record yields for Japanese sea farmers.

Pond cultures have been used for centuries for several Asian fish species, the most important of which is the common freshwater carp. In 1965, the last year for which figures are available, about 2 million tons of this fish were raised in mainland China. Usually the fish spawn and the young are reared in huge ponds. Development is improved by fertilizer additions, such as egg yolk paste, rice bran, peanut cake, or small aquatic animals. Often the ponds are located on farmlands near a pig sty, which provides nutrients for the developing fish. Unlike most other fish, carp are hardy in captivity and grow rapidly, often being large enough to market in about six months. They provide an important source of protein for the Chinese people.

Two other important cultivated fish are tilapia and milkfish. Tilapia, first cultured by the ancient Egyptians, is essentially a fresh-water fish. It spawns readily in ponds, and most species reproduce so well that over-population is a problem. Most common in Java and Japan, tilapia culture has spread to many African countries, where it is usually the most important fish eaten. Milkfish are one of the few ocean fish to be successfully pond-cultured. They will not spawn in captivity, however, so the prospective farmer must go out and catch the young fish, which are then put in the pond and reared to maturity. Indonesia and Taiwan have had extensive experience with milkfish culture.

The average productivity of aquaculture is quite high when compared to that of other methods of producing animal protein (see Table 11.2). Since the F.A.O. has estimated that the area devoted to aquaculture can be increased greatly, it represents an important potential source of food. One expert, Dr. J. Bardach, feels that the present annual production of 4 million tons of fish and shellfish could be increased tenfold.

The U.S. Navy is currently studying the possibility of using aquaculture to produce large amounts of plants. The plants in question, giant brown algae called kelp, would be grown on floating booms in the open ocean. Mineral nutrition for the kelp would be provided by mechanically agitating the water to produce an upwelling. The kelp, grown in huge floating farms, would be harvested by ships and processed on the spot into carbohydrate-based foods and feeds. A pilot project is underway, and, if it is successful, a 100,000-acre kelp farm should be in operation by 1985.

Table 11.2 Production of animal proteins, in tons per square kilometer per year.

Method	Yield
Cattle on pasture land	2 to 80
Free-swimming fish	6 to 17
Anchovies (Peru)	440
Carp culture (China)	750
Oyster culture (Japan)	3,000

ADVANCES IN FOOD TECHNOLOGY

The aims of agriculture are to increase the quantity and improve the nutritional quality of people's food. A major problem with the quality of food is that many people subsist on a diet whose protein content is inadequate or inappropriate. A major problem with the quantity of food is that the rising demand for meat in the developed areas has put great pressure on the grain-production capacities of many countries. As a result, grain is being used for animal feed rather than for human food. Food technology is developing to the point where it can make an important contribution to the solution of these problems.

Fortification

Fortification is the addition of nutrients to a food that is deficient in them. In 1947, beriberi was common in the Philippine province of Bataan because the people were eating polished rice as a staple. The rice germ, rich in vitamin B_1, is removed when rice is polished during milling. The provincial government fortified the rice by adding the vitamin at the mill, and, four years later, the incidence of beriberi was reduced by 69 percent. In an adjacent province where rice was not fortified, the incidence of the disease increased during that period. Currently, rice is fortified with vitamins in many countries. In many developed countries, white wheat flour, which is deficient in several vitamins and in the amino acid lysine, is fortified with these substances and sold as "enriched" flour. In India, a Dutch chemical firm provides bakeries with a mixture of lysine and vitamins, and the "Modern Bread" that is made is possibly the most nutritious sold anywhere in the world.

Fortification has several advantages as a method of improving nutrition. It is inexpensive: the cost of fortifying the major cereal grains with the appropriate vitamins, minerals, and amino acids would add approximately 10 percent to the wholesale cost of the grain. This is very little compared with the cost of other methods of improving dietary protein, especially the cost of eating meat. Fortification requires no special marketing costs or altered food preparation, since the product is largely unchanged. Fortification is also a relatively fast way to improve nutrition. The results of a decision to fortify a food reach the people immediately, in comparison with the long lead times needed for innovations in plant breeding.

A disadvantage of fortification is that its costs are recurring: the extra chemicals must be added to the food each time it is processed. Nutritional improvement by means of plant breeding, in contrast, does not have recurring costs; once the new strain is developed, it can be used from then on. A second, and more serious, drawback to fortification schemes is that they only benefit those consumers who buy their food commercially. Although almost all people in the developed countries purchase salt (with added iodine) at the market, only 20 percent of the rice eaters in Bangladash buy rice at the market; the remainder grow their own or buy from the grower. In India, the cost of fortifying 100 million loaves of "Modern Bread" is only $100,000 per year. But over $2 million are spent annually on promotion to get the people to buy the bread. The U.S. Agency for International Development is currently studying three cases of fortification: wheat in Tunisia, rice in Thailand, and corn in Guatemala. The logistics of the process, its cost, and its effects on community nutrition are being closely monitored. This study will provide valuable data for evaluating the potential efficacy of proposed fortification schemes.

Processing

About one-quarter of the total fish catch is now used to manufacture fish meal for use as animal feed. Some of the meal comes from by-products of fish that is processed for other purposes, and the remainder of the meal derives from whole fish, such as the anchovy. A process has been developed by which much of these fish products destined for meal can be converted into a protein-rich flour for human use. The fish or fish products are steam-cooked and squeezed to remove water and fats. The resulting flour, the fish-protein concentrate, can be used to make bread, soups, pastes, and so on. The fish generally used, hake from South America, yields a flour that is 75 percent protein by weight, and the protein contains adequate levels of all amino acids. A major problem with fish flour has been consumer acceptability. Tests in Chile of bread made from increasing amounts of the flour revealed that most people could detect an objectionable fishy odor in the bread when the fish-flour concentration was as low as 3 percent. In the U.S., the Food and Drug Administration severely restricted use of the concentrate because products made from it were "esthetically unacceptable." More recently, this restriction has been released as technology has improved to the point where consumer acceptance is predicted. Tests of the accept-ability of fish-concentrate food are underway in South America and Asia.

Throughout the underdeveloped regions, soybeans, cottonseed, and peanuts are used extensively for their oils. After the oil has been squeezed out of the seeds, the residues are rich in protein, and an estimated 20 million tons of protein is produced each year in this manner. Unfortunately, little of this protein has been used for human consumption. One problem is that the consistency of soybean flour is poor for cooking. Recently, food tech-nologists have improved soy flour by compounding it with corn meal and milk solids. This mixture has then been liquified and sold in Asia as a nu-tritious beverage, Vitasoy. In Latin America, the mixture has been pressed into cakes and sold as Incaparina. In addition, soybean grits are now widely used as a breakfast cereal.

The residues of peanut seeds after processing for oil are over 35 percent protein, and can supply 1.6 million tons of protein to India each year. They are being used as a supplement to wheat flour, and have also been pressed into palatable cakes called Provita. These cakes are being used as a diet supplement for school children. Peanut solids can be made into a dried, "milk-like" powder. In India, because of the poor condition of livestock, milk is in chronically inadequate supply; "peanut milk" could be a valuable substitute.

Cottonseed residues after oil extraction are over 50 percent protein, but contain gossypol, a substance poisonous to humans. Recently, scientists at the U.S.D.A. developed a technique for physically separating out the gossypol from the protein. Flour developed from this process is 70 percent protein. Over 5 million tons of cottonseed protein are produced worldwide each year, and over 80 percent of this production is in the underdeveloped countries. A pilot plant at Hubli, in southern India, has been producing cottonseed flour since 1970, and a large-scale plant is now operating in Lubbock, Texas. These developments indicate that cottonseed protein will be important for human nutrition in the future.

Animal-Product Analogs

One way to reduce the consumption of meat and meat products is to replace them with plant products which look and taste like the animal meat products. Margarine, usually a product of vegetable oils, is produced as an analog of animal-derived butter, and now outsells the latter in many countries. Cooking oils and shortenings derived from plants have replaced animal fats, such as lard. Plant-derived products are replacing cream and whipping cream. As a result of these changes, the U.S. now has only half the number of dairy cows that it had in 1940. However, meat consumption has doubled in this period. Food chemists have now turned their attention to using plant products to replace meat.

Meat analogs made from plant products have several advantages over meat. The analog is cheaper to produce, both in cash outlay and in terms of the world grain resources. In the U.S. in 1976, one pound of ground beef cost 30 percent more than a pound of soybean beef analog. Another advantage of the meat analogs is that their nutritional value can be carefully controlled during manufacture. Fortification, for example, is easily carried out. Finally, meat analogs often need no refrigeration, and can have a long stability on the shelf in factories and markets. This considerably reduces marketing costs.

Three types of processes are used to make meat analogs from plant products. The first is to heat mixtures of wheat, soy, and milk solids, which are then formed into frankfurters or bologna. A second method is to make an aqueous paste from soybean protein, wheat, oils, and flavors, and to heat the mixture to form a gel; this is then used as a spread for sandwiches. The third, and most recent, method was developed in 1954 by R. Boyer from the technology of the textile industry. A soy-protein mass is forced through a membrane with tiny holes, and the streamlets that emerge are coagulated in an acid bath and stretched into thin fibers. These fibers can be coated with fats, vitamins, minerals, colorings, and flavorings. Amino acids (soybean protein is deficient in methionine) are also added at this stage. The coated fibers are then bound together and formed into a marketable product (see Figure 11.2).

The resulting meat analog is usually 30 to 60 percent protein, and in nutritional composition is identical to or superior to its meat counterpart. In a study made in Guatemala, meat analogs were indistinguishable from beef in promoting growth and maintaining health in young rats, dogs, and children. Although too expensive for use in the underdeveloped countries, meat analogs are being widely used in the rich countries, and will doubtless lead to a lowering of meat consumption. The U.S.D.A. in 1972 predicted that 20 percent of all processed meat consumed in the U.S. will be replaced by soybean-based meat analogs by 1980.

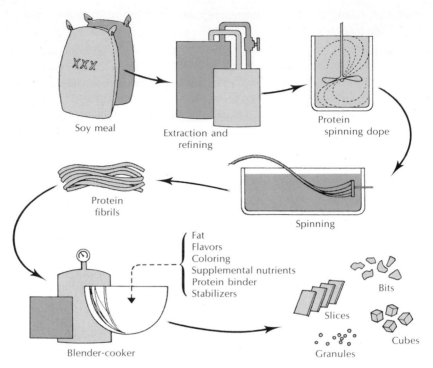

FIGURE 11.2
Making soybean protein into meat analogs. (From R. Mateles and S. Tannenbaum, Single-Cell Protein. MIT Press, 1968, p. 373.)

NOVEL FOOD SOURCES

Leaf Protein

Although leaves are not rich in protein, leaf protein is the world's largest source of readily obtainable protein. Humans cannot derive much nutrition by eating most leaves directly, because they cannot digest the cellulose-rich walls of the leaf cells. The young and tender leaves of some vegetables are the only exceptions to this general rule. However, if leaves are crushed in water, the leaf proteins can be separated out and processed into a cellulose-free powder called leaf-protein concentrate. Currently leaf-protein concentrate is being used only as an animal feed, because its green color (due to the chlorophyll) makes it look unpalatable to many people.

Table 11.3. Comparison of yields from corn and from a cassava and leaf-protein system.[a]

Crop	Yield in kilograms			Protein/carbohydrate ratio
	Carbohydrate	Protein	Total	
Corn (1.0 hectare)	2,000	300	2,300	1:7
Cassava (0.8 hectare)	6,920	–	7,920	1:7
Leaves (0.2 hectare)	–	1,000		

[a]From J. T. Worgan, "World Supplies of Proteins from Unconventional Sources."

A plant at Brawley, California, operated by Batley-Janss Enterprises, is turning out ten tons of protein feed from alfalfa leaves per day. A similar plant went into operation in 1974 in Hungary. Most of the early work on developing large-scale methods to extract leaf proteins were carried out in Great Britain by Prof. N. W. Pirie. In 1974, U.S.D.A. scientists developed a technique which results in a colorless, tasteless powder containing over 95 percent protein. Tests are underway to evaluate its effectiveness as a fortification in beverages.

If edible leaf protein can be produced on a large scale, it could have a significant impact on human nutrition. Yields of 25 tons of protein per hectare have been reported for wheat and barley leaves. Frequent and judicious harvesting of leaves for protein could leave sufficient leaves on the plant for a high yield of grain, yet provide additional protein which would otherwise be lost. Another proposal is to plant two crops: a high-yielding traditional crop and a leafy one for protein harvest. These possibilities are outlined in Table 11.3. Cassava is grown as a high-yielding, carbohydrate-rich crop. Part of the land is set aside for a leafy crop from which protein is extracted. As a result, much more food is produced than would be produced by an identical area planted with corn, and the quality of the food produced in both systems is identical.

Single-Cell Protein

Microorganisms such as bacteria, yeasts, and algae have several attractions as a potential source of dietary protein. They grow rapidly, producing a biomass that is at least 50 percent protein in dry weight. They convert a high proportion (75 percent) of the nitrogen supplied in their growth medium into cell protein; in agriculture, the conversion rate of applied nitrogen fertilizer to plant protein is lower. The microbes produce proteins that are adequate in lysine, the amino acid commonly deficient in human diets, and so the proteins may be used as a dietary supplement. Finally, microbial growth is free of the limitations of climate and land.

Different species of microbes can use different sources of chemical energy for growth. The single-celled algae can photosynthesize, and hence can use solar energy. In Japan, pilot plants have been set up for algal culture on large circular ponds, 0.2 hectares in surface area. The net productivity of such a pond is 200 tons of organic matter per hectare per year. When compared with the growth of land plants, this yield is rather modest. However, the cultures yield 30 times as much protein as a bean crop, and the algal protein is of superior nutritional quality.

Many species of yeasts and bacteria can use hydrocarbons, molecules composed of hydrogen and carbon only, as an energy source. Petroleum consists largely of hydrocarbons, and there is much interest in the potential use of oil or oil by-products to produce protein-rich concentrates. Since the late 1960's, British Petroleum has operated a plant capable of producing 20,000 tons of protein per year. In this plant, 100 tons of hydrocarbons yield 50 tons of yeast protein. The yeast cells use the wax fraction of petroleum, which accounts for only 2 percent of the crude oil and is a by-product of the refining process. If this wax fraction from all the petroleum produced worldwide in a given year were used in such plants, a vast amount of protein could be produced. In 1970, for example, world petroleum production was 2,300 million tons; 2 percent of this amount, 46 million tons of hydrocarbons, if used to grow yeast, could yield 23 million tons of yeast protein, close to the total amount of protein needed by the human race for that year! Currently, protein from petroleum is not being produced on such a grand scale. One problem is high cost. Another is that certain substances in petroleum are toxic to man; these can get into the yeast cells, rendering them useless as food. Finally, there is great consumer resistance to eating "petro-protein," as was demonstrated in 1976, when British Petroleum had to close down plants in Europe and Japan because of consumer resistance.

A third, promising energy source for production of single-cell protein is carbohydrate. Many microbes can grow by using cellulose, a molecule indigestible by man and hence a by-product of conventional agriculture. Wheat straw and maize cobs are currently converted to protein by using them as animal feeds, but they could produce protein more efficiently if used as "food" for microorganisms. Although less microbial protein is produced from a ton of carbohydrate than from a ton of hydrocarbons, the limited global reserves and rising prices for the hydrocarbons make carbohydrates a much more likely source for the future. The duPont Company in the U.S. has a pilot plant that grows fungi on molasses, beans, or cassava, and the protein produced can easily be converted into meat analogs. However, the process is far from being commercially feasible yet, and considerable research remains to be done on it.

CHAPTER 12 Conclusion: The Prospects

Too many people are hungry. Can the Earth produce enough food to feed these hungry people and the millions who are added each year?

The intensive application of science to crop production that culminated in the green revolution represents an impressive achievement. Crop yields have increased, and over-all world food production has increased by an average rate of 2.4 percent per year for the last two decades. Unfortunately, this rate of increase is only slightly above the population growth rate. Thus the amount of food produced per person has only increased by 0.2 percent per year. Presumably, even this slight increase means a better diet for all in a world where the food-people balance is precarious. But the social, political, and economic systems have been slow to distribute the fruits of the new agricultural technologies. Whereas per-capita increases in food production in the developed countries have averaged 1.5 percent annually for the last two decades, the figure for the underdeveloped countries has been 0.1 percent (see Figure 12.1). Thus the green revolution in the under-developed countries has allowed them to keep food production up with population growth. But there has been little real improvement in the diets of millions who are in chronic nutritional need.

Population projections make it clear that, even if birth control measures were instituted immediately, the Earth's human population would increase by several billion during the next 50 years (Table 1.3). Continuing pressure on the world's food resources is therefore a major problem facing mankind, and it has been the source of much debate among politicians and scientists. This debate has been characterized by much uncertainty, because the rate of population growth, the availability and efficacy of fertilizers and pesticides, the cost of energy, the weather, the progress of agricultural

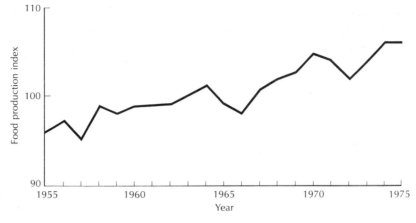

FIGURE 12.1.
Food production per person, worldwide, 1955–1974. The numbers are relative amounts, with 1963 = 100. (Data from F.A.O.)

research, and outbreaks of major crop diseases cannot be accurately pre-dicted. Nevertheless, decisions must be made, using the available informa-tion, and it is the task of policymakers to make informed guesses about the future of the world food problem.

Starting from the same (or at least similar) statistics, various scientists have reached diametrically opposed conclusions about the future of the food-population balance. Some feel that the battle to feed the world's hungry is over, and are pessimistic about the ultimate outcome. Paul Ehrlich, a Stanford University professor, said: "Those clowns who are talking of feeding a big population in the year 2000 from make-believe 'green revo-lutions' should learn some elementary biology, meteorology, agricultural economics, and anthropology." William Paddock, a consultant on tropical development, wrote that the potential of the current green revolution is too limited to provide a solution to the population problem. Other scientists are optimistic, feeling that the recent (1972) setbacks in agricultural pro-duction were due to temporary factors. Lester Brown, an agricultural econ-omist, has projected a hopeful agricultural future as a result of the green revolution. He wrote in 1970 that "these new seeds may affect the well-being of more people in a shorter period of time than any other technological advance in history." Roger Revelle, director of the Center for Population Studies at Harvard University, wrote in 1974: "There is no simple and dramatic formula for drawing back from the precipice. An obvious, difficult, but in the long run absolutely essential step is to reduce rates of population growth. Meanwhile, food supplies can be increased along three lines of action: in the short run, creation of a world food bank; in the long run, modernization of agriculture in the underdeveloped countries; and finally, a sharp intensification of agricultural and food research."

This debate among scientists has, not surprisingly, been reflected by a similar debate among politicians. At the world population conference in 1974, several representatives from the developed countries proposed broad plans for population control in the underdeveloped countries. The latter responded negatively to these suggestions, demanding instead a re-distribution of the wealth of the richer nations to support their expanding populations. At the world food conference in 1974, the underdeveloped countries demanded extensive, immediate food aid, as well as increased technological assistance from the developed nations. They received instead only promises from the richer nations, as well as threats that food aid may be contingent upon the poor countries' making their natural resources avail-able for use by the rich. With the economic difficulties of the developed countries in the mid-1970's, it is not surprising that politicians have taken a nationalistic view of the world food problem.

Solution of the world food problem is urgent. Most proposed solutions fall into one of three policy alternatives. The first is "business as usual." Its advocates propose no massive schemes of foreign aid and no alteration in living standards in the developed countries. Their hope lies in a techno-logical solution: perhaps all the food needed in the world can be obtained from single cells or from some not-yet-discovered chemical synthesis pro-cess. Perhaps these processes could indeed feed 15 billion people with no adverse effects on the environment. Technology has wrought miracles before, and, its advocates suggest, can solve the food problem. Technological optimism has strong political appeal, since it promises more of the same and gradual social change. The situation is analogous to the one faced by many of the developed countries following the oil embargo in 1974: faced with limited supplies of oil, the U.S. could have drastically altered its life-style to be less dependent on it; instead, a technological solution—looking for domestic oil and other energy sources—was adopted.

The second alternative proposes that the limits of food production have been reached, and that there are already too many people on earth. Any attempt to feed even those now present, let alone the foreseen extra billions, will inevitably lead to environmental disaster because of fertilizer, pesticide, and water pollution. In addition, the attempt to feed the under-developed world will deplete the Earth's resources so much that the resource supply for all people will be inadequate. Therefore, advocates of this alternative propose taking a careful inventory of the capacities of the earth, estimating an optimal population, and letting the "excess" people starve. This viewpoint has been most lucidly stated by ecologist Garrett Hardin in his concept of "lifeboat ethics." Hardin defines the earth as a lifeboat, or series of lifeboats, which are occupied by the developed nations. The metaphor envisages the hungry two-thirds of the world as people in the water who must be prevented from getting into the boat lest everyone, rich and poor, drown. Preventing the poor nations from "getting into the boat" of development requires a fundamental change in the morality of many of the developed nations. The moral principle of generosity has guided the aid policies of the rich nations until now. In the future, advocates of this alternative suggest, a new morality—that of custodianship of the human race—should prevail.

The third alternative acknowledges that the Earth has a finite ability to support people, but proposes that this limit to growth has not yet been reached. The disasters and world-wide famines forecast for the coming decades by the advocates of the second alternative can be avoided if we vigorously proceed along four lines. First, effective birth control must be instituted everywhere, but especially in the developing countries, so that population growth will be reduced and the human population will be stabilized. Second, we must make every possible attempt to increase crop production, especially in the developing countries. This can be done by promoting the green revolution so that its potential can be reached. Both the large farmer and the smaller, more traditional farmer must be provided with the necessary inputs to maximize food production. Agriculture, say the proponents of this position, can be carried out in a manner which will damage the environment less than it has in some areas of the world. New strains, new agricultural systems, new methods of pest control, and new approaches to providing crop plants with the necessary nutrients will allow people to increase crop production without irreparable damage to the environment. Third, the developed countries must reduce their waste of the world's resources. Scarce and increasingly costly mineral and energy reserves are too often used to produce convenience items, whereas they should be used for food production.

Finally, this alternative requires that the developing countries vigorously pursue their industrial development without neglecting their agricultural development. This may be the most difficult goal to attain. Rising incomes and higher standards of living generally mean better diets and less children, because people have money to buy food and the motivation to have smaller families. Development in the poor countries often bypasses two large groups of people: the urban unemployed and the rural poor. Creating jobs for these people and raising their living standard could have a direct effect on the population problem. When Europe and North America were developing rapidly in the nineteenth century, the unemployed rural poor flocked to the cities, where a labor-intensive industry was expanding. Virtually all those who had left the land found jobs. A similar movement is now taking place in the developing countries, but the conditions are different. Urbanization in some developing countries is proceeding very rapidly—major urban centers are doubling in size every ten years—but what little industry there is is often capital-intensive and not labor-intensive. Most of those who flock to the cities do not find jobs. The resulting situation is highly unstable, even potentially explosive; so various international agencies, such as the World Bank, are encouraging those types of investment that will benefit the poor. All of these developments—population stabilization, increased food production, restriction of wasteful use of resources, and industrial development—must be pursued vigorously and immediately if this alternative is to succeed. The efforts made by agricultural scientists are doomed to failure unless the human population is stabilized.

The decision between these alternatives has not yet been made. At the U.N.-sponsored food and population conferences in 1974, many underdeveloped countries made a plea for adoption of the third alternative. But almost passively, the developed countries seemed to take the first position. In the meantime, an increasing number of scientists are publicly advocating the second alternative. In the world today, no problem of this magnitude can be local. The food problem affects all people, and it is time for mankind to deal with it.

Further Reading

CHAPTER 1

Ecoscience: Population, Resources, Environment, by P. Ehrlich, A. H. Ehrlich, and J. Holdren. W. H. Freeman and Company, 1977. One of the best books dealing with the impact of population growth and technological progress on the Earth's resources and the environment.

Famine, 1975! by W. Paddock and P. Paddock. Little, Brown, 1967. An analysis of the world food crisis which concludes that the developed countries must decide who will starve among the underdeveloped countries.

"The Human Population." *Scientific American,* September 1974. An entire issue devoted to aspects of the human population, its origins, and its increase.

The Hungry Planet, by G. Borgstrom. Macmillan, 1965. One of the first books to bring to the attention of a large segment of the public that the population explosion will soon outstrip food production.

In the Human Interest, by L. Brown. Norton, 1974. An analysis of the limits of the food-producing capacity of the Earth and a rationale for population controls.

The Limits to Growth, by D. Meadows, D. Meadows, J. Randers, and W. Behrens. Universe, 1972. A computerized projection of the future which predicts that, with current trends, the population death rate will increase during the next century.

Man and His Environment: Food, by L. R. Brown and G. Finsterbusch. Harper and Row, 1972. An account of various aspects of food production, food consumption, agricultural development, and the green revolution.

Resources and Man. Committee on Man, National Academy of Sciences—National Research Council. W. H. Freeman and Company, 1969. A collection of articles on the future availability of our most important resources.

World Food Resources, by G. Borgstrom. Intext, 1973. A description of the production and consumption of food in the world.

CHAPTER 2

Energy and Protein Requirements. F.A.O., 1973. A report by experts on human nutritional requirements, written in nontechnical language.

Food: Readings from Scientific American, complied by J. Hoff and J. Janick. W. H. Freeman and Company, 1973. Many excellent articles on nutrition and food production.

Hunger, U.S.A. Beacon Press, 1968. A report by the Citizens' Board of Inquiry into hunger and malnutrition in the United States.

The Malnourished Mind, by E. A. Shneour. Doubleday, 1974. A provocative paperback which explores all the available evidence about the effect of malnutrition on learning abilities.

Man and Food, by M. Pyke. World, 1973. Contains basic information on the nutritive values of foods.

Nutrition, by M. S. Chaney and M. L. Ross. Houghton-Mifflin, 1971. An up-to-date treatment of the principles of human nutrition.

Nutritional Studies. F.A.O., 1953-1972. Nine detailed reports on various foods, such as wheat, corn, and milk.

Principles of Food Science, by G. Borgstrom. Macmillan, 1968. Two volumes covering food chemistry, preservation, marketing, and nutrition.

U.S. Nutrition Policies in the Seventies, edited by Jean Mayer. W. H. Freeman and Company, 1973. A shortened version of the reports of The White House Conference on Food, Nutrition, and Health held in 1969.

CHAPTER 3

Biology of Plants by P. H. Raven, R. F. Evert, and H. Curtis. Worth, 2d ed., 1976.

Botany, by T. E. Weier, C. R. Stocking, and M. G. Barbour. Wiley, 1970.

Botany, by C. L. Wilson, W. E. Loomis, and T. A. Steeves. Holt, Rinehart, and Winston, 1971.

Botany: An Ecological Approach, by W. A. Jensen and B. F. Salisbury. Wadsworth, 1972. These four are just a few examples of excellent basic botany textbooks which cover many areas of botany in some detail.

Cereal Crops, by W. Leonard and J. Martin. Macmillan 1963. An excellent, readable summary of all aspects of producing these crops.

The Oxford Book of Food Plants, by G. B. Masefield, M. Wallis, S. G. Harrison, and J. B. E. Nicholson. Oxford University Press, 1969. A beautifully illustrated book on mankind's food plants.

Plant Science: An Introduction to World Crops, by J. Janick, R. Schery, F. Woods, and V. Ruttan. W. H. Freeman and Company, 2d ed., 1974. A comprehensive text on crop-plant physiology and its relation to production.

Plants and Civilization, by H. G. Baker. Wadsworth, 1965. A short account of the most important plants used by people.

Plants for Man, by R. W. Schery. Prentice-Hall, 2d ed., 1972. An account of many economically important plants, not only those used for food.

Rice and Man, by L. Hanks. Aldine-Atherton, 1972. A treatment of rice cultivation from an ecological point of view.

"Soybeans," by F. Dovring. *Scientific American,* February 1974, p. 14. A short article about the economic importance of soybeans for U.S. agriculture and trade.

Wheat in Human Nutrition, by W. R. Aykroyd and J. Doughty. F.A.O., 1970. A short book about the nutritional value of wheat and wheat-derived foods and the production and uses of wheat.

CHAPTER 4

"Agricultural Productivity," by R. S. Loomis, W. A. Williams, and A. E. Hall. *Annual Review of Plant Physiology,* 22 (1971), 431–468. A summary of research carried out by many investigators on this important subject.

The Challenge of Ecology, by C. L. Kucera, V. V. Mosby, 1973. There are many basic textbooks in ecology that discuss many ecological principles, including food chains, energy transfer, and fluctuations in natural population, as well as other ecological problems that we discuss in this book.

CO$_2$ Metabolism and Plant Productivity, edited by R. Burris and C. Black. University Park Press, 1976. A collection of articles by leading scientists on the theory and practice of improving plant productivity.

Concepts of Ecology, by E. J. Kormondy. Prentice-Hall, 1969.

Fundamentals of Ecology, by E. P. Odum. W. B. Saunders, 1971.

Introduction to Crop Physiology, by F. L. Milthrope and J. Moorby. Cambridge University Press, 1974. In this paperback, the physiology of plants is discussed in terms of its significance for crop productivity.

The Living Plant, by P. Ray. Holt, Rinehart, and Winston, 1969. An excellent and concise treatment of plant physiology, including photosynthesis and water relations. Photosynthesis is also discussed in the botany textbooks listed in the additional readings for Chapter 3.

The Mechanism of Photosynthesis, by C. P. Wittingham. American Elsevier, 1974. An extensive, technical discussion of many aspects of photosynthesis.

Photosynthesis, Photorespiration, and Plant Productivity, by I. Zelitch. Academic Press, 1971. A summary of research on photosynthesis and photorespiration, most of it done by the author.

"The Upper Limit of Crop Yield," by J. Bonner. *Science,* 137 (1962), 11–15. A somewhat technical discussion of the subject.

CHAPTER 5

The Biosphere: Readings from Scientific American. W. H. Freeman and Company, 1970. A book of readings from *Scientific American* dealing with energy, mineral, and food resources in the biosphere, including discussions of the nitrogen cycle, the carbon cycle, and mineral cycles.

"Chemical Fertilizers," by C. Pratt. *Scientific American,* June 1965. Describes the manufacture and use of inorganic fertilizers.

Diagnosis of Mineral Deficiencies in Plants. Her Majesty's Stationery Office, 1951. A manual of plant diseases and their manifestations.

Eutrophication: Causes, Consequences, Correctives, by J. W. Bigger and R. B. Corey. National Academy of Sciences, 1969.

Life in the Soil, by R. M. Jackson and F. Raw. St. Martin's Press, 1966. A short paperback about soil organisms and the methods used to study them.

Mineral Nutrition of Plants: Principles and Perspectives, by E. Epstein. Wiley, 1972. A textbook about all aspects of mineral nutrition of plants written by a man who has devoted his entire life to scientific research on this problem.

The Nature and Properties of Soil, By H. O. Buckman and K. C. Brady. Macmillan, 1969. A basic textbook about soils and plant growth.

"Nutrient Cycling," by H. Bormann, F. H. Likens, and G. E. Likens. *Science,* 155 (1967), 424–429. A discussion of the movement of plant nutrients in the ecosystem.

Plant-Water Relationships, by R. O. Slatyer. Academic Press, 1967. An excellent textbook about the subject.

Soil Conditions and Plant Growth, by E. W. Russell. Longmans, Green, 1961. One of the standard textbooks about plants and soils, especially concerning crop production and farming practices, including crop rotations and manuring.

"Zero-Tillage," by K. Baeumer and W. A. P. Bakermans. *Advances in Agronomy,* 25 (1973), 77–123. An article about the current agricultural practice of tilling the soil as little as possible.

CHAPTER 6

"Agricultural Centers and Non-Centers," by J. Harlan. *Science,* 174 (1971), 468–474. A discussion of the theory that agriculture originated not only in distinct centers but also in vast geographical regions.

The Domestication and Exploitation of Plants and Animals, edited by P. J. Ucko and G. W. Dimbledy. Aldine, 1969. A collection of original research papers by some 50 scientists dealing with many aspects of domestication. An excellent source book.

"Domestication of Corn," by P. C. Mangelsdorf, R. S. MacNeish, and W. C. Galinat. *Science,* 143 (1964), 538–545.

Eat Not This Flesh, by F. J. Simoons. University of Wisconsin Press, 1961. A discussion of the origins of food taboos.

"The Ecology of Early Food Production in Mesopotamia," by K. V. Flannery. *Science,* 147 (1965), 1247–1256. An account of the emergence of agriculture in this area of southwestern Asia.

"Origin of the Common Bean, *Phaseolus vulgaris,*" by H. S. Gentry. *Economic Botany,* 23 (1969), 55–69.

Prehistoric Agriculture, edited by S. Struever. Doubleday, 1970. A collection of papers dealing with the origin of agriculture, the consequence of the agricultural transition, and the role of agriculture in the development of civilizations.

Seed to Civilization: The Story of Man's Food, by C. B. Heiser. W. H. Freeman and Company, 1973. An excellent, crop-by-crop account of agricultural origins, and of the role which various crops play in the human diet.

Seeds, Spades, Hearths, and Herds: The Domestication of Animals and Food-stuffs, by C. O. Sauer. The MIT Press, 1969. Originally written in 1952, this book does not take into account the more recent information about domestication, but is nevertheless a very stimulating discussion of agricultural origins.

"Some Considerations of Early Plant Domestication," by C. B. Heiser. *Bioscience,* 19 (1969), 228–231. A discussion of the ecological principles which underlie plant domestication.

"Toxic Substances in Plants and the Food Habits of Early Man," by A. C. Leopold and R. Ardrey. *Science,* 176 (1972), 512–513. A brief article about toxic substances in food and the effect of cooking on these substances.

"Wheat," by P. C. Mangelsdorf. *Scientific American,* July 1953, pp. 2–11.

CHAPTER 7

"Agricultural Potential of the Tropics," by J. H. Chang. *The Geographical Review,* 58 (1968), 333–351. A discussion of the limits of agricultural production in the humid tropics.

"Control of the Water Cycle," by J. Peixoto and M. Kettani. *Scientific American,* April 1973, pp. 56–61. A clear summary of the global uses of water.

"Desalination," by R. Probstein. *American Scientist,* 61 (1973), 280–293. A fairly technical but concise statement of this field, with numerous examples.

Fertilizer Industry Series, published by the U.N. Industrial Development Organization (1972–1975). A series of studies on the sources, uses, and economics of fertilizers.

Human Ecology, by P. Ehrlich, A. Ehrlich, and J. Holdren. W. H. Freeman and Company, 1973. A book written for nonscientists about human impact on the environment; includes many references to agriculture.

"Lateritic Soils," by M. McNeil. *Scientific American*, November 1964, pp. 96–102. A discussion of the properties of lateritic soils and the problems encountered in the agricultural usage of lateritic soils.

Losing Ground: Environmental Stress and World Food Prospects, by E. Eckholm. Norton, 1976. An analysis of the effects of intensive agriculture and forestry on the environment.

Starvation of Plenty? by Colin Clark. Taplinger, 1970. A summary of the technology of high-yield agriculture.

Survey of Multiple Cropping in Less-Developed Nations, by D. Dalrymple. U.S.D.A. Foreign Economic Service, 1971.

World Geography of Irrigation, by L. Cantor. Praeger, 1970. A readable description of the methods and effects of irrigation.

"World Outlook for Conventional Agriculture," by L. Brown. *Science*, 158 (1967), 604–611. Discusses the limits of high-yield technology.

CHAPTER 8

Advances in Agronomy. This annual volume has summaries of many current topics in agricultural research. Articles of interest on pest control include "Behavior of pesticides in soils" (in volume 23, 1971), and "Resistance of plants to insects" and "Behavior of herbicides in plants" (in volume 24, 1972).

"Agricultural Pest Control and the Environment," by G. W. Irving, Jr. *Science*, 168 (1970), 1419–1424.

Biological Control, by R. van den Bosch and P. Messenger. Intext, 1973. An excellent, concise treatment of the subject, emphasizing insects.

Effects of Herbicides in South Vietnam. National Academy of Sciences, 1974. An exhaustive report on all aspects of this use of herbicides, including their effects on humans.

Herbicide Handbook of the Weed Science Society of America. Humphrey Press, 1970. A list of the chemistry, use, and actions of all herbicides.

"Insect Control: Alternatives to the Use of Conventional Pesticides," by R. W. Holcomb. *Science*, 168 (1970), 456–459.

Mode of Action of Herbicides, by F. M. Ashton and A. S. Crafts. Wiley-Interscience, 1973. A textbook about the mode of action of the many herbicides presently used in the U.S.

Pest Control: Strategies for the Future. U.S. National Academy of Sciences, 1972. A readable, nontechnical summary written by experts.

Pesticides and the Living Landscape, by R. L. Rudd. University of Wisconsin Press, 1964. A survey of the various kinds of chemical pesticides and their effects on the environment.

Plant Pathology, by G. Agrios. Academic Press, 1972. A survey of fungal and microbial diseases.

Silent Spring, by Rachel Carson. Houghton Mifflin, 1962. The first book to bring the dangers of extensive pesticide use to the attention of a large segment of the American public.

"Third-Generation Pesticides," by C. Williams. *Scientific American,* July 1967, pp. 13–17. Describes the isolation and use of hormones for insect pest control.

"Toxic Substances and Ecological Cycles," by G. M. Woodwell. *Scientific American,* March 1967, pp. 24–31. Describes the accumulation of toxic substances as they move up the food chain.

CHAPTER 9

Agricultural Genetics, by J. Brewbaker. Prentice-Hall, 1964. A good treatment of the principles of heredity as applied to breeding systems.

"Agriculture in China," by S. Wortman. *Scientific American,* June 1975, pp. 13–21. An account of the green revolution by a member of a U.S. team that visited China in 1974.

Ceres. A biomonthly publication of the F.A.O. Written for the layman, articles describe current progress in world agriculture.

"Farm Crops of China," by P. Kung. *World Crops,* 1975. A series of articles examining in detail agricultural practices in China.

"Plant Germ Plasm Now and For Tomorrow," by J. L. Creech and L. P. Reitz. *Advances* in *Agronomy,* 23 (1971), 1–50. A scholarly account about the need to collect a great variety of plant strains to insure that they will be available to future plant breeders.

Seeds of Change, by L. Brown. Praeger, 1970. Describes the background of plant breeding and the green-revolution strains of wheat and rice.

"Triticale," by J. Hulse and D. Spurgeon. *Scientific American,* August 1974, pp. 72–80. An excellent description of the breeding and potential usefulness of this wheat-rye hybrid.

CHAPTER 10

All in a Grain of Rice, by G. Castillo. Southeast Asia Regional Center of Research in Agriculture, 1976. A comprehensive review of the introduction, effects, and prognosis of the green revolution in the Philippines.

"Bringing the Green Revolution to the Shifting Cultivator," by D. Greenland. *Science,* 190 (1975), 841–844. Describes work in Nigeria.

Focal Points, by G. Borgstrom. Macmillan, 1973. Presents a generally pessimistic analysis of the green revolution.

Food, Population, and Employment: Impact of the Green Revolution, edited by T. Poleman and D. Freebairn. Praeger, 1973. Contains papers on the economic and social impact of the green revolution.

Giant in the Earth, by R. Katz. Stein and Day, 1973. A popularized and optimistic account of the green revolution.

Green Revolution, by S. Johnson. Harper and Row, 1972. In travelogue style, a description of the human aspects of high-yield agriculture in the underdeveloped regions.

Green Revolution, by M. S. Randhawa. Wiley, 1974. An account of successes in the Punjab of India, written by one of the architects of India's green revolution.

In the Human Interest, by L. Brown. Northon, 1974. An analysis of the limits of food production and a rationale for population control.

The Nutrition Factor, by A. Berg. Brookings, 1973. An examination of progress and proposals in meeting nutritional needs in the underdeveloped countries.

Politics of World Hunger, by P. Simon and A. Simon. Harper and Row, 1973. An excellent treatment of development assistance.

Race Between Population and Food Supply in Latin America, by T. Lynn Smith. University of New Mexico Press, 1976. The social effects of agriculture and its progress from Mexico to Chile, by an experienced observer.

Reaching the Developing World's Small Farmers, by C. Streeter. Rockefeller, 1973. Describes the Puebla and numerous other projects.

Studies on the Green Revolution, U.N. Research Institute for Social Development, Geneva. A series of five studies encompassing the scientific, economic, and social aspects of the green revolution.

"World Food Prices and the Poor," by L. Schertz. *Foreign Affairs,* 52 (1974), 511-537. An analysis of the economics of the world food problem.

CHAPTER 11

Aquaculture, by J. Bardach, J. Ryther, and W. McLarney. Wiley, 1972. A comprehensive treatment of the subject.

"Food from the Sea," by W. E. Ricker, in *Resources and Man.* W. H. Freeman and Company, 1969.

"Food Resources in the Ocean," by S. Holt. *Scientific American,* September 1969, pp. 178-194. A readable summary of the methods of fishing.

"Leaf Protein as a Human Food," by N. W. Pirie. *Science,* 152 (1966), 1701-1705.

New Protein Foods, edited by A. Altschul. Academic Press, 1974. Contains numerous articles on fortification and novel food sources.

"Photosynthesis and Food Production in the Sea," by J. H. Ryther. *Science,* 166 (1969), 72-80.

"Protein from Petroleum," by A. Champagnat. *Scientific American,* October 1965, pp. 13-17. A popular article by one of the pioneers in this field.

Review and Comparative Analysis of Oilseed Raw Materials and Processes Suitable for the Production of Protein Products for Human Consumption. U.N. Industrial Development Org., 1974. A concise summary of the vast unused protein resources in oilseeds.

Sea Against Hunger, by C. P. Idyll. Crowell, 1970. An optimistic view of the potential of the ocean to produce food.

Third International Conference on Food Science and Technology. Institute of Food Technologists, 1971. Contains many papers on new food sources.

CHAPTER 12

Food: Politics, Economics, Nutrition, and Research, edited by P. Abelson. AAAS, 1975. A compendium of articles on the world food problem by authorities in their fields.

Genesis Strategy, by S. Schneider and L. Mesirow. Plenum, 1976. Discusses the effects of climatic change on world agriculture and human survival.

The Limits to Growth, by D. Meadows, D. Meadows, J. Randers, and W. Behrens. Universe, 1972. The computerized world model from the Club of Rome.

"Living on a Lifeboat," by G. Hardin. *BioScience,* 24 (1974), 561–563.

Mankind at the Turning Point, by M. Mesarovic and E. Pestel. Dutton, 1974. A second Club of Rome Study, more optimistic in its conclusions.

"Relevance of Demographic Transition Theory to the Developing Countries," by M. Teitelbaum. *Science,* 188 (1975), 420–428. Compares the current situation in the developing countries with that of North America and Europe in the nineteenth century.

"Tragedy of the Commons," by G. Hardin. *Science,* 162 (1968), 1243–1248. A lucid statement of the third alternative.

Units of Measurement

To convert item in column 1 to that in column 2, multiply by:	Column 1	Column 2	To convert item in column 2 to that in column 1, multiply by:
	Length		
0.621	kilometer (km)	mile (mi.)	1.609
1.094	meter (m)	yard (yd.)	0.914
	Area		
0.386	square kilometer (km²)	square mile (mi.²)	2.590
247.1	square kilometer	acre	0.004
2.471	hectare (ha)	acre	0.405
	Mass		
1.102	metric ton	ton	0.907
2.205	kilogram (kg)	pound (lb.)	0.454
	Yield		
0.446	tons per hectare	tons per acre	2.240
0.891	kg per ha	lb per acre	1.121

APPENDIX II

Glossary

Adsorption. The adhesion of ions or molecules to a solid surface—such as a soil particle—resulting in a higher concentration of the adsorbed substance.

Aleurone layer. The outer layer of the endosperm of a cereal grain; usually rich in protein, vitamins, and minerals.

Algae. Simple plants that mostly live in water. They range in size from single cells to giant seaweeds, and do not contain xylem or phloem cells.

Amino acid. An organic molecule that is the building block of proteins; contains carbon, hydrogen, oxygen, nitrogen, and sometimes sulfur.

Anion. A negatively charged ion.

Aquaculture. "Sea farming": containment and mass rearing of animals or plants that live in water.

Asexual propagation. Propagation that does not depend on the union of specialized reproductive cells; common in plants such as strawberries.

Autotroph. An organism which can make its own food from chemically simple precursors; green plants are autotrophs, for example.

Auxin. A plant hormone that regulates many aspects of plant growth and development, including cell elongation, apical dominance, and fruitset.

Biological control. The use of natural enemies to reduce the numbers of a pest.

Calorie. The amount of heat energy that raises the temperature of one gram of water by one degree centigrade; 1,000 of these calories make up one nutritional "calorie."

Carbohydrate. A class of organic molecules that contain carbon, hydrogen, and oxygen, usually in a 1:2:1 ratio; sugars, starch, and cellulose are examples.

Carnivore. An animal that feeds on other animals; lions, birds of prey, and trout are examples.

Carpel. The female reproductive organ of the flower; a carpel is a modified leaf which carries the ovules within it.

Carrying capacity. The maximum number of a given organism that can be supported by a given environment.

Cation. A positively charged ion.

Cellulose. A large molecule consisting of a long chain of glucose sugar units; found in plant cell walls.

Cell membrane. The outer limiting membrane of a cell which surrounds the entire protoplasm.

Cell wall. A rigid, cellulose-containing layer that surrounds a plant cell.

Chloroplast. The structure where photosynthesis occurs within green plant cells.

Chromosomes. The bodies or structures in the nucleus of the cell which contain the genes; genes are arranged linearly along the length of the chromosome.

Coenzyme. An organic molecule which helps an enzyme carry out its function.

Consumer. An organism which uses dead or living organic matter as food; humans are an example.

Cytokinins. A group of plant hormones that regulate cell division, organ formation, and leaf senescence.

Decomposer. An organism that uses dead organic matter as food, returning it to the environment as simple substances.

Demography. The study of human populations.

Diffusion. The process whereby molecules become uniformly distributed in a defined system.

Ecosystem. The sum total of the interacting biological and physical factors in a defined area.

Endosperm. Food-storage tissue contained within many seeds.

Enzyme. A protein molecule capable of speeding up a biochemical reaction without itself being changed by the reaction.

Ethylene. A plant hormone involved in fruit ripening, flower fading, leaf fall, and other processes.

Eutrophication. Mineral enrichment of water that leads to abundant plant growth.

Evapotranspiration. The loss of water from the soil by direct evaporation and by transpiration through the plants.

Fallow. Land that is normally used for farming and is left unseeded for one or more growing seasons.

Feed. Food supplied by man to domesticated animals.

Food chain. A chain of organisms in a natural community; each link in the chain feeds on the one below and is eaten by the one above; the autotrophs are at the bottom, the largest carnivores at the top.

Fruitwall. A matured, ripened ovary (or group of ovaries) containing the seeds; can be thick and fleshy, as in our edible fruits, but also hard and dry, as in cereal grains.

Gene. A discrete unit of inheritance that gives an organism the potential to have a specific trait.

Germ. As in wheatgerm; the embryonic root and shoot in a seed.

Gibberellins. A group of plant hormones which regulate many aspects of plant growth and development, including cell elongation, flowering in some plants, and use of the endosperm in cereal seedlings.

Grain. The fruit of a cereal; consists of a seed and a hard, thin fruitwall.

Herbivore. An animal that feeds on plants.

Heterotroph. An organism that feeds on other organisms because it cannot make its own food from simple molecules; humans are an example.

Heterozygous. Having two different forms of a particular gene.

Homozygous. Having two identical forms of a particular gene.

Horizon. A distinct layer of soil; many soils have three horizons which differ in the extent to which the parent rock has been broken down.

Hormone. A molecule which is produced in very small amounts in one part of an organism and travels to another part where it has a specific effect.

Humus. Decomposing organic matter in the soil.

Hybrid. An organism that is the result of the reproductive union of two different genetic strains.

Hydrogenation. Treatment of unsaturated fats to make them saturated; it causes the conversion of an oil to a fat.

Hydrologic cycle. The continuous cycling of water between the oceans, air, and land.

Ion. An electrically charged atom or group of atoms; positively charged ones are *cations,* and negatively charged ones are *anions.*

Kwashiorkor. A protein deficiency disease; it often develops when a child is weaned, and its diet is changed from mother's milk to food that is rich in sugar and starch.

Laterite. A hard, permanent crust that develops on many tropical soils after they are directly exposed to the sun and air.

Legumes. A group of plants which includes beans, clover, and peas.

Lipid. An organic molecule, containing carbon, hydrogen, and oxygen, that is insoluble in water; fats and oils are examples.

Lysine. One of the eight amino acids that humans must ingest in their diet; present only in low amounts in cereal grains.

Marasmus. A protein and calorie deficiency disease; occurs when people are undernourished.

Meiosis. The two successive divisions of the nucleus which cause the chromosome number of the cell to be halved; sex cells are produced as a result of meiosis.

Meristem. Region of a plant where a cell division occurs.

Metabolism. The sum total of all chemical reactions that occur in an organism.

Microbe. Microscopic organisms; bacteria are an example.

Mitosis. A process during which all the chromosomes in a cell divide lengthwise and give rise to two identical sets of chromosomes.

Mutation. A sudden, permanent, and inherited change in a gene.

Mycorrhiza. A symbiotic relationship between soil fungi and the roots of certain plants.

Nematode. A type of worm, often found in soils, that can cause plant diseases, and transmit numerous human diseases.

Nitrogen fixation. The conversion of nitrogen gas to ammonia; occurs in bacteria and certain algae.

Nucleus. A specialized structure in the cell which contains all the chromosomes; not found in bacterial cells.

Organic molecules. Molecules that contain carbon atoms; often used to mean molecules from living organisms.

Ovule. The structure containing the female reproductive cell of a plant, the egg.

Parenchyma cells. Large, thin-walled cells which carry out many of the important functions of the plant (e.g., photosynthesis and food storage).

Pest. An organism that noticeably damages humans or their domesticated animals and plants.

Pesticide. A chemical that kills a pest.

Petal. A flower part, usually conspicuously colored.

Phenotype. The inherited traits that are manifested in an organism; the result of the interactions of genes and environment.

Pheromone. A molecule used for communication between organisms of the same species.

Phloem. Plant tissue that conducts organic molecules, such as sugars and hormones, from one plant part to another.

Photoperiod. The relative durations of light and darkness in a 24-hour period.

Photorespiration. A light-stimulated process, chemically distinct from respiration, in which plants respire away much of the carbon dioxide that has been fixed in organic molecules.

Photosynthesis. The chemical reactions wherein plants use sunlight, water, and carbon dioxide to form glucose and oxygen.

Plankton. Single-celled or small multicellular organisms that live in water.

Pollen. Spherical structures which contain the male reproductive cells of most crop plants that reproduce sexually.

Polyploids. Plants which have more than two complete sets of chromosomes in each cell.

Producer. An organism that uses photosyntehsis to convert solar energy into biochemical energy.

Productivity. The rate at which energy is stored as matter in an organism or ecosystem.

Protein. A long chain of amino acids linked together.

Protoplasm. Living material of an organism.

Respiration. The breakdown of sugars, within an organism, with concurrent release of energy.

Runner. A stem which grows horizontally along the ground and may send down roots to form a new plant.

Saturated bond. A linkage between two carbon atoms involving a single covalent bond.

Sepal. A flower part, often green; encloses the flower bud before it opens.

Silt. Fine soil particles which are carried by moving waters and deposited as a sediment.

Species. A group of organisms which have distinctive characteristics and which cannot breed with any other group of organisms.

Spike. A cluster of flowers on an elongated stem, as in wheat.

Stamen. The male reproductive organ of a flower; it produces pollen.

Stomate. An opening in the leaf which can be closed and opened, and through which water vapor and other gases are exchanged between leaf and atmosphere; most leaves have thousands of stomates.

Symbiosis. The relationship between two species which is of mutual benefit; bacteria living inside legume roots are an example.

Tilth. The structure or crumbliness of a soil; refers to the degree to which individual soil particles stick together and form larger aggregates.

Tissue. A group of cells performing the same function.

Transpiration. The loss of water from the leaves of a plant as a result of the evaporation of cellular water and the movement of water vapor through the stomates.

Trophic level. A step occupied by a particular kind of organism in a food chain.

Tubers. Enlarged, short, fleshy underground stem, such as that of a potato.

Vitamin. An organic molecule required in small amounts by an organism because it cannot synthesize the molecule.

Weed. A plant which grows in a cultivated area to the detriment of the desired cultivated plant.

Xylem. Plant tissue that conducts water and dissolved minerals from one plant part to another.

Index

INDEX